EVOLUTIONARY EATING STYLE

Achieving Health and Sustainability through Conscious Habits

Carlos Silva

CONTENTS

Title Page

Preface

1.   Introduction: The Journey towards Health and Well-being   1

2.   The Mind and Body: Nourishing Yourself with Wisdom   14

3.   The Crucial Moment at the Supermarket: Conscious Choices   39

4. Unraveling Labels: The Art of Understanding What We Eat   51

5. The Grain Revolution: Understanding the Impact of Wheat and Cereals on Health   69

6. The Magic of Insulin: Unveiling the Secret of Weight Regulation and Glycemic Control   84

7. The Power of Fasting: Renewing the Body and Mind   94

8. The Low Carb Universe: Exploring the Wonders of the Ketogenic and Low Carb Diet   109

9. Moving with Purpose: Simple Routine of Exercises and Everyday Activities   170

10. Small Choices, Big Results: Transforming Habits and Lifestyle   187

11. The Art of Personalization: Building Your Own Dietary Style   197

PREFACE

Tired of diets that don't work and empty promises to achieve the health and well-being you deserve? We present to you our book: "Evolutionary Eating: Achieving Health and Sustainability with Conscious Habits"! In this book, we unravel the secrets behind conscious and balanced eating, guiding you on a journey of self-discovery and transformation. Throughout the pages, you will find valuable information about the relationship between food and brain health, the importance of understanding food labels, the impact of grains on health, and much more.

Explore the world of low-carb and intermittent fasting, learn to personalize your own eating style, and discover how small choices can lead to significant results. Additionally, we provide a 4-week weight loss program to put conscious eating into practice, helping you achieve your health and well-being goals.

With practical tips and delicious recipes, "Evolutionary Eating" will help you transform your habits and achieve the health and sustainability you have always dreamed of. Whether you are a beginner in healthy eating or someone who is already familiar with the subject, this book is a valuable resource for anyone seeking a more balanced and healthy life.

Don't waste any more time! Join us on this incredible journey towards an evolutionary and conscious eating stylc, and discover how to achieve health and sustainability with conscious habits. Get your copy now and transform your life for the better!

1. INTRODUCTION: THE JOURNEY TOWARDS HEALTH AND WELL-BEING

1.1. Contextualizing the Current Health Scenario

We live in an era of constant technological advancements and social changes, where global connections and the availability of information deeply and rapidly impact our lives. While these transformations have brought many benefits, such as access to a wide variety of foods and improvements in medicine, we also face a series of challenges related to health and well-being.

The statistics are concerning: the prevalence of obesity, type 2 diabetes, cardiovascular diseases, and certain types of cancer is increasing. Simultaneously, mental disorders such as depression, anxiety, and chronic stress have become more common, affecting the quality of life of millions of people worldwide.

Faced with this reality, it is essential for us to reconsider our daily habits and choices, especially regarding nutrition and lifestyle. Our dietary decisions have a direct impact on our physical, mental, and emotional health. Therefore, it is crucial to adopt a more conscious and balanced approach to our diet and daily habits.

This book aims to assist you on this transformative journey. We will address the key aspects of mindful eating and how it can contribute to achieving a healthier and more balanced life. With a perspective grounded in evidence and real-life experiences, you will discover how to make informed decisions and gradually adapt your dietary and lifestyle habits to achieve the balance and well-being you aspire to.

Together, we will embark on this journey with courage

and determination, moving towards a healthier and more conscious lifestyle. Every choice matters, and every step brings us closer to our ultimate goal: the health and balance of our body, mind, and spirit.

1.2. The need for mindful eating

In a world full of food options and conflicting information, it is essential to adopt a mindful approach to our eating. But what does it truly mean to be mindful when choosing the foods we consume? It involves acquiring knowledge about what we ingest, paying attention to our choices, and understanding the impact of those decisions on our health and well-being.

Opting for mindful eating begins with seeking information. When we know the nutrients present in foods, their beneficial effects, and potential health risks, we can make more suitable and balanced choices. This way, we can adjust our diet to our personal needs and goals, enjoying a healthier and more fulfilling life.

Moreover, the mindful approach encourages us to listen to the signals from our bodies. Learning to identify sensations of hunger and satiety, understanding how different foods affect us, and adapting our diet to our energy demands are fundamental aspects of this practice.

In this book, we will explore various elements of mindful eating and how to apply them in your daily life. We will discuss topics such as understanding nutrients and their effects, the connection between food and health, the importance of developing balanced habits, and much more.

Throughout this journey, you will realize that mindful eating goes beyond simply choosing healthier alternatives. It is a path of self-discovery and self-awareness, allowing the development of a more harmonious and balanced relationship with food and oneself. After all, when we nourish ourselves mindfully, we nurture not only our bodies but also our minds and spirits.

1.3. Challenges and overcoming them: How to start the transformation

Embarking on the journey of transforming towards a low-carb and non-industrialized lifestyle can be challenging, especially when old habits are hard to let go of. However, with determination and a gradual approach, it is possible to overcome obstacles and implement significant changes that align with your everyday life.

Imagine yourself on a trail, walking towards a healthier lifestyle. The first step in this journey is to acknowledge the eating patterns you want to change. Perhaps you want to reduce carbohydrate consumption, eliminate processed foods, or incorporate more natural and fresh foods into your diet.

Now, set realistic and achievable goals. Like a traveler who chooses the less steep and safer path, be patient and avoid radical changes that may be difficult to sustain. Focus on small achievements, and remember that every step taken in the right direction is a victory.

It is important to acquire basic knowledge about the principles of the low-carb and ketogenic diet, as well as the benefits of a non-industrialized diet. With a solid foundation of information, you will have the confidence to create your own balanced lifestyle, including nutrition and exercise.

Develop a resilient and flexible mindset to face the challenges of this journey. Imagine yourself as a tree that adapts to climate changes, growing stronger with every storm it faces. In times of difficulty, remember why you decided to follow this path and use these challenges as opportunities for learning and growth.

Lastly, seek support and share your experiences with others who are walking similar paths. Connecting with friends, family, or support groups can be a valuable source of motivation and encouragement, helping you stay firm in your pursuit of a healthy and balanced lifestyle in harmony with your daily tasks.

1.4. Target audience: Who is this book for

This book was created with the everyday people in mind, those who face a busy routine, balancing work, family, responsibilities, and leisure time. If you find yourself caught in the whirlwind of modern life, held hostage by the food industry, and struggling to find time and motivation to take care of yourself, this book is for you. Together, let's embark on the path to a healthier and more balanced life, with a focus on mindful eating and overall well-being.

Imagine yourselves as sailors in an ocean of temptations, navigating the currents of daily life, facing storms of stress and anxiety. This book is like a lighthouse that illuminates the way to the safe harbor of health and happiness, guiding you in the right direction and helping you avoid hidden dangers.

This book is perfect for:

1. *Everyday warriors:* Those who face the daily battles of work, family, and responsibilities but seek a balance between life's demands and self-care.

2. *Survivors of the food industry:* People who wish to escape the grip of processed and industrialized foods and regain control over their food choices by adopting healthier and more mindful habits.

3. *Adventurers in pursuit of well-being:* Those who are willing to explore new territories, facing challenges and overcoming obstacles to achieve a healthier and fulfilling life.

4. *Builders of meaningful connections:* People who wish to strengthen relationships with friends and family, enjoying moments of leisure and happiness, and sharing accomplishments on the journey towards health and well-being.

5. *Life transformers:* Individuals who are ready to embrace change and break paradigms, reinventing themselves and creating a new lifestyle that reflects their true aspirations and values.

Join us on this journey and discover how this book can light the way to a healthier and happier life, filled with mindful choices and rewarding moments. This is your invitation to join us in this adventure, where we are all the heroes of our own stories.

1.5. Reframing the relationship with food

Our relationship with food is an essential part of our lives and often goes from being a source of nourishment and pleasure to becoming a stressful and confusing aspect. This book aims to help you reframe your relationship with food, transforming it into a healthy, rewarding, and mindful experience.

1. Demystifying myths and beliefs: It is important to debunk myths and misconceptions about food so that we can understand the true value and role of food in our lives. Throughout this journey, we will address common misconceptions and provide evidence-based information to help you make informed decisions about your diet.

2. Establishing a healthy emotional connection: Food should not only be a source of nutrients but also of pleasure and satisfaction. We will work to help you develop a healthy emotional relationship with food, cultivating the habit of savoring each meal as if it were a symphony of flavors, and recognizing the role that food plays in our emotional and social lives.

3. Focus on quality, not quantity: We believe that the key to mindful eating is prioritizing the quality of the foods we consume, treating them as precious treasures for our bodies, rather than simply counting calories or restricting portions. By learning to choose fresh, nutritious, and minimally processed foods, you will be taking an important step towards improving your relationship with food.

4. Food as self-care: A fundamental part of reframing the relationship with food is recognizing that taking care of the body and mind through the choice of healthy foods is a form of self-care, as if you were planting seeds of well-being in a personal garden. This book encourages you to consider food as a way to nourish and take care of yourself, promoting well-being in all aspects of life.

5. Flexibility and balance: Lastly, we want you to understand that mindful eating does not mean rigidity or deprivation, but rather finding the perfect balance, like a tightrope walker on their wire. It is possible to enjoy special moments without feeling guilty or overly restrictive. The key is to learn to make healthy choices that fit your lifestyle, without losing sight of the pleasure and joy that food can bring.

By reframing the relationship with food, we hope you will feel more confident, healthy, and happy, finding joy and balance in your food choices, and positively transforming your life with every bite.

1.6. The importance of balance in the diet

In the pursuit of a healthy and balanced life, diet plays a crucial role. Just as the famous quote from the Swiss-German physician and physicist Paracelsus in the 16th century said, "The dose makes the poison," balance in the diet is crucial to ensure well-being.

A balanced diet is like a mosaic of colors and flavors, where the variety of foods ensures the supply of essential nutrients for the proper functioning of our bodies. The approach advocated in this book seeks this balance through the choice of natural and minimally processed foods, avoiding excessive consumption of carbohydrates and processed products.

Each nutrient has a specific role in our bodies, like musicians in an orchestra. Proteins, carbohydrates, fats, vitamins, and minerals work together to keep our vital functions in harmony. With this approach, you provide your body with the appropriate amount of these nutrients, ensuring that it functions efficiently and healthily.

It is important to remember that balance in the diet is not a one-size-fits-all formula. Each person is unique, with their own nutritional needs, preferences, and life circumstances. This book will help you find the "right dose" for your needs, allowing for moments of discipline and others that are more relaxed, balancing rigor and flexibility.

In this way, you will no longer be a hostage to industrialized food, but you will also not become a prisoner of a diet filled with restrictions and fears. Avoiding extremes is crucial. Extremely restrictive diets are rarely sustainable or beneficial in the long term, like a pendulum swinging violently from one side to the other. Moderation is the key to avoiding excesses and deficiencies that can harm our well-being.

Learning to listen to your body is a crucial aspect of this journey. The human body is an incredibly intelligent machine, capable of providing us with signals and feedback about its needs. By learning to interpret these messages, you can adjust your diet according to your body's needs, finding the perfect balance, like a sailor adjusting the sails to the wind.

By understanding and applying the concept of balance in the diet, you are taking an important step towards improving your health and quality of life. This book will serve as a guide and a beacon, illuminating the path to a healthier and happier life through mindful and balanced food choices.

1.7. The journey of self-discovery and self-awareness.

The journey of self-discovery and self-awareness is an essential component in transforming your relationship with food and adopting a more balanced lifestyle. Throughout this adventure, you will be invited to dive into your inner world, observing patterns of thoughts, feelings, and behaviors that influence your food choices.

Imagine yourself as an explorer, venturing into new territories of self-knowledge and unraveling the secrets that your own body and mind hold. In this process, you will learn to identify signals of hunger, satiety, and emotional cravings, enabling you to make more mindful choices aligned with your true needs.

It is not just about changing how you eat but also transforming how you see yourself and relate to yourself. Self-acceptance and self-love are fundamental elements in creating an environment conducive to change, where guilt and self-criticism are replaced by understanding and compassion.

On this journey, you will discover that the path to a more balanced and healthy life also involves the heart and mind, and that self-awareness is a powerful ally in the pursuit of holistic well-being. And remember: with each step on this journey, you will be building a better and more authentic version of yourself every day, reflecting in all aspects of your life.

2.   THE MIND AND BODY: NOURISHING YOURSELF WITH WISDOM

2.1. The relationship between nutrition and brain health

Navigating through the waters of knowledge, we discover that the brain, a majestic beacon of wisdom, is strongly affected by the food we consume. The quality and quantity of these nutrients determine whether our brain will be a fortress of health and well-being or a shipwreck, ravaged by storms of neurological diseases.

Sugar, as enticing as the sirens' song, is one of the main villains in the story of brain health. Scientific studies, such as the one conducted by Lustig et al. (2012), reveal that excessive sugar consumption is linked to brain inflammation, increased insulin resistance, and a higher risk of neurodegenerative diseases. Type 3 diabetes, a form of Alzheimer's associated with insulin resistance in the brain, is a sad example of this relationship (de la Monte & Wands, 2008).

On the other hand, the ketogenic diet stands as a protective shield against the harmful effects of sugar and brain inflammation. A study published by Croteau et al. (2018) demonstrates that the ketogenic diet can reduce inflammation in the brain and prevent the development of neurological diseases such as Alzheimer's and Parkinson's. Another research conducted by Paoli et al. (2013) shows that this diet can also reduce the production of free radicals, unstable molecules that attack our brain and contribute to the development of these illnesses.

The available statistical data highlights the urgency to change our dietary paradigm. According to the World Health Organization (WHO), nearly 50 million people worldwide suffer from dementia, with Alzheimer's disease responsible for

60-70% of these cases. The prevalence of type 2 diabetes also continues to increase globally, with over 422 million people affected in 2014 (WHO, 2016).

Real-life cases illustrate the power of dietary change in transforming lives. The American author and podcaster Jimmy Moore is an inspiring example: after adopting the ketogenic diet, he lost over 100 kilograms and completely reversed his type 2 diabetes. Another touching story is that of Anna, a 40-year-old lawyer who regained her ability to concentrate, memory, and quality of sleep by giving up fast food and sugary treats.

In summary, the diet we choose is the roadmap we chart for our brain's journey. The ketogenic diet and other low-carb approaches serve as compasses that guide us towards a healthier future filled with cognitive vitality. Meanwhile, excessive consumption of processed foods, sugar, and carbohydrates is like a threatening iceberg, jeopardizing the integrity of our precious brain ship.

2.2. The key nutrients for the brain and body

Continuing through the waters of knowledge, it is crucial to understand the essential nutrients that fuel the symphony of our brain and body. These are the foundations that build and sustain our inner fortress, allowing the orchestra of neurons to play in perfect harmony.

Diving into the depths of scientific studies, we discover that the key nutrients for the brain and body are crucial for a healthy and vibrant life. A study conducted by the Academy of Nutrition and Dietetics (2012) points to a series of key nutrients that promote health and well-being, particularly for older adults.

Among the essential nutrients, protein stands out as the guardian of our cellular structure and function. It is indispensable for tissue repair and growth, neurotransmitter and hormone synthesis, and immune system balance. Protein can be found in foods such as meat, fish, eggs, dairy, legumes, and nuts.

B vitamins, such as B6, B9 (folate), and B12, are the beacons that illuminate cognition and nervous system health. These vitamins play a critical role in energy production, neurotransmitter synthesis, and maintenance of the integrity of brain cells. Foods like fish, poultry, eggs, dairy, and leafy green vegetables are rich sources of these vitamins (Mahan et al., 2012).

Another essential nutrient is omega-3, the trade winds that calm inflammation and sustain brain function. Eicosapentaenoic acid (EPA) and docosahexaenoic acid (DHA), found in fatty fish such as salmon and sardines, are crucial for the development and maintenance of brain cells and communication between them (Swanson et al., 2012).

Minerals also play their heroic role in this story. Magnesium, for example, is a silent maestro responsible for over 300 biochemical reactions in the body, including neurotransmitter synthesis and maintenance of cognitive function. Foods like spinach, avocado, nuts, and seeds are excellent sources of magnesium.

In summary, the key nutrients for the brain and body form a united team, working together to sustain and protect our health. Proteins, B vitamins, omega-3, and minerals are true navigators, guiding us toward a horizon of well-being and vitality. By choosing the right foods, we are capable of orchestrating a symphony of health and happiness in our lives, ensuring a fulfilling and rewarding journey.

2.3. Beneficial and harmful foods to health

In our journey towards healthy eating, it is important to know the foods that can elevate our body and mind to new heights, as well as those that can bring us down. In this chapter, we will explore 10 beneficial and 10 harmful foods to health, revealing their nutritional and caloric secrets, as well as their relationship with disease prevention or development.

Imagine that our body is a garden and each food is a seed. Beneficial foods are seeds that blossom into health and vitality, while harmful ones germinate disease and discomfort. Let's dive into the universe of these seeds and discover which ones to plant and which ones to avoid in our garden of life.

Beneficial Foods:

1. Eggs (especially the yolk): Nutrients - protein, vitamin B12, vitamin D, choline; Calories - 143 kcal/100g. They are crucial for brain function and immune system strengthening.

2. Beef liver: Nutrients - vitamin A, vitamin B12, iron, copper; Calories - 135 kcal/100g. Assists in the formation of blood cells and prevents anemia.

3. Grass-fed beef: Nutrients - protein, vitamin B12, iron, zinc; Calories - 250 kcal/100g. Promotes muscle health and strengthens the immune system.

4. Sardines: Nutrients - omega-3, vitamin D, calcium; Calories - 208 kcal/100g. Reduces the risk of heart disease and improves brain function.

5. Coconut: Nutrients - healthy fats, vitamin C, iron; Calories - 354 kcal/100g. Strengthens the immune system and improves skin and hair health.

6. Nuts and seeds (almonds, walnuts, chia seeds, flaxseeds): Nutrients - omega-3 fatty acids, magnesium, vitamin E, antioxidants; Calories - 576 kcal/100g (almonds), 654 kcal/100g (walnuts), 486 kcal/100g (chia seeds), 534 kcal/100g (flaxseeds). Promote cardiovascular and cognitive health.

7. Berries (blueberries, strawberries, raspberries): Nutrients - antioxidants, vitamin C, fiber; Calories - 57 kcal/100g (blueberries), 32 kcal/100g (strawberries), 52 kcal/100g (raspberries). Aid in the prevention of cardiovascular and neurodegenerative diseases.

8. Extra virgin olive oil: Nutrients - healthy fats, vitamin E, polyphenols; Calories - 884 kcal/100g. Protects the heart and combats inflammation.

9. Broccoli: Nutrients - vitamin C, vitamin K, folic acid, sulforaphane; Calories - 34 kcal/100g. Assists in cancer prevention and strengthens the immune system.

10. Spinach: Nutrients - vitamin A, vitamin C, vitamin K, iron, magnesium; Calories - 23 kcal/100g. Promotes eye health and strengthens bones and muscles.

Now, let's turn our attention to harmful foods, those that, like weeds, threaten the balance and harmony of our garden.

1. Industrialized vegetable oils: Calories - 884 kcal/100g. Rich in omega-6 fats, which, in excess, can cause inflammation and increase the risk of heart disease.

2. Sugar: Calories - 387 kcal/100g. Contributes to obesity, type 2 diabetes, heart disease, and premature aging.

3. Bread: Calories - 266 kcal/100g (white). Can cause spikes in blood sugar, leading to an increased risk of type 2 diabetes and obesity.

4. Soy: Calories - 173 kcal/100g (cooked). Can interfere with thyroid function and affect the absorption of essential nutrients when consumed in excess.

5. Pizza: Calories - 266 kcal/100g (medium). Rich in saturated fats and sodium, contributes to the risk of heart disease and high blood pressure.

6. Ultra-processed deli meats: Calories - 330 kcal/100g (average). Contain additives, sodium, and nitrates associated with a higher risk of cancer and heart disease.

7. Soft drinks: Calories - 42 kcal/100g. High in sugars and chemical additives, contributes to obesity, diabetes, and cardiovascular diseases.

8. Alcohol: Calories - 7 kcal/g. Excessive alcohol consumption increases the risk of liver diseases, cancer, and heart problems.

9. Pasta: Calories - 157 kcal/100g (cooked). Can cause spikes in blood sugar and contribute to an increased risk of type 2 diabetes and obesity, especially when consumed in excess.

10. Wheat flour: Calories - 364 kcal/100g. Can cause inflammation and digestive problems, as well as contribute to obesity and heart disease.

By nurturing our garden with beneficial seeds, we cultivate a life full of health and well-being. On the other hand, by planting harmful seeds, we risk harvesting disease and discomfort. The choice is ours, and with wisdom and discernment, we can enjoy a flourishing and vibrant garden where health and happiness intertwine harmoniously.

When selecting the foods we consume, it is important to remember that we are the gardeners of our bodies and minds. Investing in beneficial foods is like watering and fertilizing the soil, providing the ideal environment for the flourishing of our health. Avoiding harmful foods, on the other hand, is like pulling out the weeds that hinder our growth and prosperity.

Throughout our journey, we may encounter temptations

and challenges, but by keeping the focus on nutrition and well-being, we will be able to create a thriving and healthy garden of life. The key lies in maintaining balance and making conscious choices, nourishing ourselves with foods that strengthen our health and avoiding those that may compromise it.

And so, with wisdom, patience, and dedication, our health and happiness will blossom, rooting us in a fertile and abundant soil where life is full and vibrant.

2.4. Eating as a means of disease prevention

The wisdom of the ancients already told us: "Let food be thy medicine and medicine be thy food." Over time, the popular saying "we are what we eat" also reinforces this idea. In a world where processed food has dominated supermarket shelves, it's as if we have forgotten these valuable lessons and distanced ourselves from the healing and preventive power of natural foods.

The prevalence of chronic diseases and weight gain has been increasing alarmingly, directly related to the adoption of diets rich in processed and ultra-processed foods. Obesity, diabetes, cardiovascular diseases, and cancer are examples of ailments associated with these dietary choices.

According to a study published in the journal "The Lancet," about 11 million deaths per year worldwide are related to poor diet. Additionally, the World Health Organization (WHO) estimates that in 2021, obesity affected over 650 million adults worldwide.

However, by reconnecting with nature and investing in minimally processed foods, we can embark on a journey of health and well-being. A clinical study called PREDIMED, published in the "New England Journal of Medicine," demonstrated that a Mediterranean diet rich in natural and minimally processed foods such as fruits, vegetables, whole grains, olive oil, and fish can significantly reduce the risk of cardiovascular events such as heart attack and stroke.

The following foods are like true magical elixirs that, when incorporated into our diet, help prevent and combat various diseases:

1. **Dark chocolate:** Improves heart health and brain

function by combating oxidative stress.

2. Berries: Aid in cellular aging prevention and the fight against chronic diseases like cancer.

3. Extra virgin olive oil: Reduces inflammation and protects the heart, preventing cardiovascular diseases.

4. Lemon: Strengthens the immune system and prevents cardiovascular diseases due to its high vitamin C content.

5. Turmeric: Aids in the prevention and treatment of chronic diseases like diabetes and cancer due to its anti-inflammatory and antioxidant properties.

6. Coconut: Improves metabolic health and has antimicrobial properties, aiding in infection prevention.

7. Eggs: Contribute to muscle, bone, and cognitive health by providing high-quality proteins and essential micronutrients.

8. Vitamin D: Essential for bone health and immune function, helping prevent autoimmune diseases and osteoporosis. The primary source of vitamin D is sunlight exposure, but it can also be found in fatty fish and eggs.

9. Apple cider vinegar: Controls blood sugar levels, reduces inflammation, and improves digestion, contributing to the prevention of type 2 diabetes.

10. Ginger: Relieves nausea, improves digestion, and reduces the risk of chronic diseases like cardiovascular diseases, thanks to its anti-inflammatory and antioxidant compounds.

Just as a gardener cares for their plants with love and attention, we must nourish our bodies with these valuable foods to strengthen our health and create a protective shield against diseases. Each food has a specific role in this mission, and by incorporating them into our diet, we will be taking care of our health and our life.

Changing our dietary habits and valuing natural and

minimally processed foods can make all the difference in the prevention and control of major diet-related diseases. By embracing this philosophy and reclaiming ancestral wisdom about the benefits of food, we are taking the reins of our well-being and building a healthier and happier future.

2.5. The Influence of Diet on Energy and Well-being

Imagine our body as a complex system of gears, where each component plays a crucial role in ensuring everything works harmoniously. In this scenario, nutrition is the oil that lubricates and keeps the gears moving. The quality of the food we consume directly affects our energy, disposition, and physical and mental well-being.

The hormone insulin, for example, plays a fundamental role in controlling energy levels. It is responsible for regulating the amount of sugar in the blood, ensuring that our cells receive enough energy to function properly. However, the old saying "the dose makes the poison" applies perfectly here: excessive or insufficient carbohydrate intake can lead to insulin resistance and fluctuations in energy levels.

It is important to remember that rates of obesity and chronic diseases have been significantly increasing worldwide. These health issues are often related to lack of energy and mental disposition. When our body is burdened with excess weight, it needs to work harder to perform simple tasks, which can lead to a vicious cycle of fatigue and lethargy.

The connection between nutrition, body, and a healthy mind is undeniable. To cultivate this harmony, we should focus on a nutrient-rich and balanced diet that promotes proper bodily function and prevents the development of insulin resistance and other diseases.

In this context, understanding the importance of balance is essential. Just like a violinist tuning their instrument, we should adjust our nutrition to find the perfect harmony among the various nutrients needed to maintain our body and mind healthy and energized.

Furthermore, it is crucial to remember that we are

complex beings, and the pursuit of energy and disposition should not be limited to nutrition alone. Practices such as physical exercise, adequate sleep, and stress management also play a fundamental role in this equation.

Like a well-tended garden, where fertile soil and proper irrigation ensure the flourishing of lush plants, our nutrition is the foundation for a fulfilling life full of energy. By nourishing our body and mind with the best ingredients, we are investing in our health, well-being, and quality of life.

Surprisingly, small changes in our dietary habits can have a significant impact on our energy and disposition. By embracing this philosophy and seeking balance between body and mind, we will be able to face the challenges of everyday life with vitality and enthusiasm.

2.6. The effects of stress and anxiety on eating: When emotions and numbers collide

In an increasingly fast-paced and challenging world, stress and anxiety have become unwanted companions in many people's lives. Studies show that the prevalence of stress and anxiety-related disorders has significantly increased in recent years. According to the World Health Organization (WHO), in 2021, depression and anxiety already affected over 322 million and 264 million people, respectively, worldwide.

These emotional problems not only impact our minds but also have direct consequences on our physical health and dietary choices. Stress and anxiety can lead to excessive consumption of processed foods that are high in sugar, fats, and chemical additives. In turn, this processed diet contributes to the rise of chronic diseases and metabolic disorders such as obesity, diabetes, and cardiovascular diseases.

A study published in the American Journal of Clinical Nutrition in 2019 revealed that the consumption of processed foods was associated with a higher risk of developing depression. This suggests that processed food not only affects our physical health but also has negative implications for our mental well-being.

To address the effects of stress and anxiety on eating habits and break this harmful cycle, it is crucial to adopt a conscious and holistic approach. We need to recognize the severity of the emotional impact on our health and seek effective strategies to cope with these emotions and make healthier food choices.

In addition to the suggestions mentioned earlier, it is important to remember that diet is just one piece of the puzzle when it comes to managing stress and anxiety. We should also invest in self-care, relaxation practices, and emotional balance, such as meditation, physical exercise, and therapy.

By tackling stress and anxiety with an integrated approach that combines healthy eating and well-being practices, we will be able to strengthen our emotional resilience and improve our physical and mental health. In doing so, we will take an important step towards a more balanced and fulfilling life.

2.7. The Role of Vitamins
and Minerals in Health

Imagine our body as a symphony orchestra in constant motion and transformation, where each component - cells, tissues, and organs - works tirelessly to ensure harmony is maintained. In this metaphor, vitamins and minerals play a crucial role, acting as silent conductors that ensure all biological functions occur efficiently and cohesively.

Vitamins and minerals are essential micronutrients, meaning our body needs them in small but regular amounts to function properly. They participate in a myriad of vital processes, from maintaining our immune defenses to energy production and hormone synthesis.

Over time, science has revealed the importance of these silent conductors, identifying more and more vital functions they perform in our bodies. Micronutrient deficiencies can lead to various health problems, from anemia and osteoporosis to weakened immune systems and neurological disorders.

A study published in The Lancet in 2018 highlighted the importance of micronutrients for global health and emphasized the need for integrated approaches to improve vitamin and mineral intake. This study reinforces the idea that ensuring adequate intake of vitamins and minerals is one of the fundamental pillars in promoting our health and well-being.

To achieve this goal, it is crucial to adopt a diet rich in fresh and minimally processed foods. By doing so, we nourish our bodies with these silent conductors, promoting our health and well-being in an increasingly challenging world.

In conclusion, do not underestimate the power of these silent conductors of our health. By paying attention to the quality and variety of the foods we consume, we can ensure that our bodies have all the necessary resources to face the challenges of daily life and maintain our health in balance.

1. Vitamin A: Essential for eye health, immune function, and reproduction. Found in foods such as carrots, pumpkin, and liver.

2. Vitamin B1 (Thiamine): Important for energy production, nerve function, and heart health. Present in whole grains, pork, and nuts.

3. Vitamin B2 (Riboflavin): Necessary for energy production, cell health, and immune system function. Found in dairy products, eggs, and dark leafy greens.

4. Vitamin B3 (Niacin): Assists in energy production, DNA synthesis, and maintenance of the nervous system. Present in meats, fish, and whole grains.

5. Vitamin B5 (Pantothenic acid): Helps with energy production, hormone synthesis, and metabolism of fats, proteins, and carbohydrates. Found in meats, eggs, and vegetables.

6. Vitamin B6 (Pyridoxine): Contributes to brain function, energy production, and red blood cell formation. Present in meats, poultry, and fish.

7. Vitamin B7 (Biotin): Necessary for skin, nail, and hair health, as well as carbohydrate, protein, and fat metabolism. Found in eggs, nuts, and legumes.

8. Vitamin B9 (Folic acid): Important for cell formation and nervous system health. Present in dark leafy greens, citrus fruits, and legumes.

9. Vitamin B12 (Cobalamin): Essential for red blood cell formation, DNA synthesis, and proper nervous system function. Found primarily in animal products such as meats, eggs, and dairy.

10. Vitamin C (Ascorbic acid): Powerful antioxidant that aids in collagen formation, iron absorption, and maintenance of the immune system. Present in citrus fruits and vegetables.

11. Vitamin D: Critical for bone health as it assists in calcium absorption and immune system regulation. We primarily obtain vitamin D through sunlight exposure but can also be found in foods such as fatty fish and eggs.

12. Vitamin E: Acts as an antioxidant, protecting cells from oxidative stress and contributing to skin and eye health. Can be found in nuts, seeds, and extra virgin olive oil.

13. Vitamin K: Important for blood clotting and bone health. Found in dark leafy green vegetables like kale and spinach, and in some non-industrialized vegetable oils such as extra virgin olive oil.

14. Calcium: Essential for bone and teeth formation and maintenance, as well as assisting in muscle function and nerve transmission. Can be found in dairy products, dark leafy greens, and fish with edible bones like sardines.

15. Iron: Necessary for red blood cell formation and oxygen transport in the blood. Present in red meats, legumes, and dark leafy greens.

16. Magnesium: Participates in over 300 enzymatic processes in the body, including energy production, protein synthesis, and muscle and nerve health. Can be found in nuts, seeds, legumes, and whole grains.

17. Zinc: Essential for immune function, DNA synthesis, wound healing, and cell growth. Found in meats, fish, oysters, and legumes.

18. Copper: Helps with energy production, collagen synthesis, and iron absorption. Found in organ meats, shellfish, nuts, and seeds.

19. Selenium: Important antioxidant that protects cells from oxidative stress and contributes to immune function. Present in Brazil nuts, fish, meats, and whole grains.

20. Iodine: Necessary for the production of

thyroid hormones, which regulate metabolism, growth, and development. Can be found in saltwater fish, dairy products, and seaweed.

2.8. The conscious consumption of proteins, carbohydrates, and fats

Imagine our body as a sophisticated engine that requires the right fuel to function efficiently. Proteins, carbohydrates, and fats are the main components of this fuel. However, the key to a healthy and balanced life is not following a restrictive diet but rather understanding and consciously choosing the foods we consume.

A more mindful nutritional approach, such as low-carb or ketogenic, helps us understand the different functions and needs of macronutrients. First and foremost, it's important to highlight that body fat and dietary fat are not the same thing. While excessive carbohydrate consumption can lead to body fat accumulation and weight gain, healthy dietary fats are essential for health and well-being.

In fact, carbohydrates are the only macronutrient that is not essential in our diet, as our body can produce the necessary energy from other sources, such as fats. This does not mean that we should completely eliminate carbohydrates but rather consciously choose those that are more nutritious and beneficial for our health.

When it comes to fats, it's crucial to distinguish between healthy fats and toxic fats. Natural fats from animal sources, such as butter, and vegetable fats, such as extra virgin olive oil, are healthy sources of energy for the body and contribute to a variety of vital functions. On the other hand, highly processed vegetable oils, such as soybean oil and corn oil, are inflammatory and can cause harm to our bodies. Several scientific studies have already demonstrated the difference between these two categories of fats and their impacts on health.

Regarding proteins, it's important to consider their bioavailability, which is the amount of protein that our body can effectively utilize. Animal protein, such as meat, has a much higher bioavailability than plant protein, such as soy. Furthermore, choosing pasture-raised animal proteins brings numerous health benefits, such as a more balanced fatty acid profile and the presence of important nutrients like vitamin K2 and conjugated linoleic acid (CLA).

Embarking on this journey towards conscious consumption of proteins, carbohydrates, and fats, it's important to remember that the key to health and balance is not restriction but rather choosing quality and nutritious foods. By fueling our "engine" with the right fuel, we are investing in our long-term health and promoting physical and mental well-being. Remember: the secret lies in making conscious and informed choices, always with the goal of achieving a healthier and balanced life.

By adopting a more conscious and informed approach to nutrition, we can find the right balance between proteins, carbohydrates, and fats that best suits our individual needs. This may include reducing the consumption of refined carbohydrates and sugars, prioritizing high-quality protein sources, and focusing on healthy fats.

The general rule is to opt for fresh, unprocessed foods consumed in their most natural state, which provide the necessary nutrients for the optimal functioning of our "engine". By paying attention to the signals of our body and adjusting our diet according to our needs and preferences, we can achieve a state of health and well-being that is sustained over time.

A useful analogy to illustrate the importance of mindful consumption of macronutrients is to think of our body as an orchestra, where each instrument plays a unique and valuable role. Proteins, carbohydrates, and fats are like the musicians of this orchestra, each contributing their own sound and harmony to create a balanced and enjoyable performance. By adjusting the quantity and quality of these "instruments," we can create a symphony of health and vitality.

Ultimately, conscious consumption of proteins, carbohydrates, and fats allows us to cultivate a healthier and more harmonious relationship with food, providing a solid foundation for a life of health, energy, and well-being. Like any journey, there may be challenges and obstacles along the way, but by committing to education and experimentation, we will discover the right path for ourselves and enjoy the lasting benefits of a balanced and healthy life.

2.9. The Importance of Vitamin D: The Sun that Illuminates Our Health

Vitamin D is often referred to as the "sunshine vitamin" due to its unique synthesis in our skin when exposed to sunlight. This nutrient is a true protagonist in the orchestra of health, playing crucial roles in numerous processes in our bodies. Further investigation into vitamin D reveals its importance in maintaining our well-being and combating diseases.

To understand how vitamin D works, it's important to know that it is not just a vitamin but also a hormone. When sunlight reaches the skin, our bodies convert cholesterol into cholecalciferol, also known as vitamin D3. This form of vitamin D is then transported to the liver and subsequently to the kidneys, where it is converted into its active form called calcitriol. Calcitriol acts as a molecular messenger, conveying important information to cells and affecting gene expression.

Proper absorption and metabolism of vitamin D depend on other micronutrients, such as magnesium, which participates in the conversion of cholecalciferol to calcitriol, and vitamin K, which works in conjunction with vitamin D to regulate calcium balance in the body.

Vitamin D plays a crucial role in bone health, aiding in calcium absorption and maintaining bone density. Furthermore, studies have shown that vitamin D possesses immunomodulatory properties, protecting against infections and autoimmune diseases. Research published in the British Medical Journal in 2017 found that vitamin D supplementation can reduce the risk of respiratory tract infections, such as the flu and colds.

Other research suggests an association between low

levels of vitamin D and an increased risk of cardiovascular diseases, type 2 diabetes, and certain types of cancer. These studies indicate the importance of maintaining adequate levels of vitamin D to preserve our long-term health.

A notable example of the importance of vitamin D in bone health is the case of astronauts. When in space, away from sunlight and the force of gravity, astronauts experience a rapid decline in bone density. The lack of sun exposure and reduced production of vitamin D in their bodies contribute to this phenomenon. NASA researchers have identified that bone loss can reach 1-2% per month during prolonged space missions, putting astronauts at risk of developing osteoporosis and increasing the likelihood of fractures.

In a low-carb/ketogenic diet, it is important to ensure adequate intake of vitamin D through foods rich in this nutrient, such as fatty fish, eggs, and liver. However, sunlight exposure remains the primary source of this vitamin.

3.   THE CRUCIAL MOMENT AT THE SUPERMARKET: CONSCIOUS CHOICES

3.1. Planning and organizing your grocery shopping

Imagine yourself as a skilled navigator, about to embark on an expedition through the vast ocean of the supermarket. Navigating the choppy waters of shelves and aisles requires planning and organizational skills, as well as the wisdom to make conscious choices.

Before setting sail on this journey, it's essential to chart a course of action and arm yourself with the perfect shopping list. Planning meals for the week and listing all the necessary ingredients can save time, money, and help avoid the temptation of buying unhealthy foods.

As you enter the supermarket labyrinth, remember that fresh and minimally processed foods are usually located in the peripheral areas of the store. Therefore, prioritize these aisles and fill your cart with high-quality vegetables, greens, meats, and dairy products.

Avoid the areas where processed and packaged foods accumulate as much as possible, as that is where the siren song of unhealthy foods can lure unprepared navigators. When confronted with a selection of products that may seem harmless, such as breakfast cereals or cereal bars, remember that many of these items can be high in sugars and refined carbohydrates, disguised under different names and appealing labels.

And speaking of labels, becoming an expert in reading labels is an indispensable skill on this adventure. Learn how to interpret the nutritional information and decipher hidden ingredients. This skill can be compared to a treasure map that reveals which foods are truly valuable for your health.

As you leave the supermarket with the treasure of healthy foods in hand, you will have taken an important step towards a healthier and more conscious life. The wise navigator's journey is a continuous learning and adaptation process, and the ability to make conscious choices while shopping is a powerful tool in your toolbox for a healthy and balanced life.

3.2. How to Avoid Traps at the Supermarket

In our journey through the supermarket maze, it's common to encounter traps and disguised temptations that can steer us away from the path of healthy eating. As experienced navigators, it's crucial to learn to identify and avoid these traps to ensure a safe route towards our ultimate goal.

Imagine the supermarket traps as treacherous islands, hiding dangers beneath the appearance of seemingly healthy and tasty foods. To navigate through these hazardous waters, follow these valuable tips:

1. Don't shop on an empty stomach: When we're hungry, we're more vulnerable to the temptation of buying unhealthy foods. Think of an empty stomach as a ship without a rudder, easily swayed by the current of sugary and carb-rich treats.

2. Focus on the periphery of the supermarket: Just like in our previous journey, stick to the store's outer aisles, where fresh and minimally processed foods tend to reside. Think of these aisles as safe routes where temptations are less likely to hide.

3. Beware of misleading labels: Many foods claim to be "healthy," "natural," or "sugar-free," but can be true traps in disguise. Learn to read and interpret labels correctly to avoid shipwrecking on an island of false promises.

4. Avoid tempting promotions: Special offers and promotions are like sirens' songs, luring the unsuspecting towards ruin. Be critical of offers and remember that a good deal may not be so good if it leads to unhealthy food choices.

5. Shop with a companion: Having a fellow traveler can help you stay focused and resist temptations. Think of a friend or family member as a navigation partner, someone to help you stay on course and face the traps together.

By following these tips and remaining vigilant, you can turn your supermarket journey into a successful and rewarding expedition. With each conscious choice you make, you're strengthening your resilience and navigation skills, becoming a true master at avoiding the traps and temptations lurking on the supermarket shelves.

3.3. The Dangers of Ultra-Processed Foods

In our quest for a healthy diet, we are often confronted with the hidden dangers of ultra-processed foods, disguised as healthy and appetizing options. As a fearless explorer, it is crucial to be vigilant and learn to identify the true threats to our health.

Imagine the world of ultra-processed foods as an ocean full of sea monsters, ready to drag us into the depths of excessive consumption of sugars, fats, and chemical additives. In addition to being traps in terms of nutritional classification, such as the Nutri-Score table, these foods can have alarming consequences for our health. Various clinical studies and scientific publications have demonstrated the link between excessive consumption of these foods and the increase in diseases such as type 1, 2, and 3 diabetes, and even cancer.

For example, a study published in the British Medical Journal (BMJ) in 2018 showed that increased consumption of ultra-processed foods is associated with a higher risk of cancer. The study followed over 100,000 adults and found that a 10% increase in the consumption of these foods was related to a 12% increase in the overall risk of cancer and an 11% increase in the risk of breast cancer.

Furthermore, statistical data has shown that the consumption of ultra-processed foods has been increasing worldwide. According to the World Health Organization (WHO), the prevalence of type 2 diabetes has increased in parallel with the expansion of consumption of these foods due to their high content of sugars, fats, and chemical additives.

To avoid the dangers of ultra-processed foods and protect our health, follow these guidelines:

1. Don't be deceived by labels: Learn to carefully analyze food labels, looking beyond the attractive Nutri-Score classifications and keywords. Remember that the true treasure lies in the ingredients and quality of the food, not just its appearance.

2. Prioritize natural and minimally processed foods: Choose foods that are closer to their natural state, such as fruits, vegetables, pasture-raised meats, and dairy products. These foods are true beacons guiding our journey towards health and well-being.

3. Avoid chemical additives and preservatives: Be mindful of artificial and potentially harmful ingredients that may be hidden in ultra-processed foods. These additives are like invisible currents, dragging us into the abyss of excessive consumption and health issues.

By following these guidelines, you will be better prepared to face the storms and traps of the world of ultra-processed foods. With knowledge and discernment, it is possible to navigate safely and confidently, leaving behind the sea monsters and embracing the true riches of a healthy and balanced diet.

With the power of conscious choices within our reach, we can explore the ocean of the food industry and find refuge in the islands of nutrition and well-being. Our journey towards health and vitality begins with every decision made in the supermarket, where we confront the treacherous waves and deceptive winds of ultra-processed foods.

Remaining alert and informed is our best defense against the traps and hidden dangers in the supermarket aisles. By prioritizing natural and minimally processed foods, analyzing labels carefully, and avoiding chemical additives and preservatives, we are navigating with a steady helm towards a healthier and fulfilling future.

So, keep honing your navigation skills, stay informed, and strengthen your determination to face the challenges. Together, we can overcome the obstacles imposed by the food industry and, with every conscious choice, build a healthier and more sustainable path for ourselves and future generations.

3.4. Identifying ultra-processed foods

Imagine the tomato as a hero in an epic saga, going through different stages of processing in its journey through the world of food. Let's follow it from its natural state to its transformation into an ultra-processed product, exploring the choices available in the supermarket and the potential health risks.

In its purest and most authentic form, the fresh tomato is a natural food, packed with nutrients and flavor. This red gem is the first stop on our journey and offers the greatest health benefits, including vitamins, minerals, and antioxidants.

Moving on in our adventure, we encounter the minimally processed tomato, such as pre-packaged fresh salads with sliced tomatoes available at the supermarket. This champion still retains many of its nutritional properties but may have undergone a process of cutting and packaging for convenience.

Next, we arrive at the realm of processed foods, where our hero transforms into tomato sauce or puree. In this form, the tomato still retains some of its nutritional value but may contain additives like salt, sugar, and preservatives to enhance flavor and shelf life.

Finally, we reach the domain of ultra-processed foods, where the tomato takes the form of ketchup. Here, the tomato loses much of its original properties, being mixed with a range of artificial ingredients such as sugars, colorings, flavorings, and preservatives.

Ultra-processed foods represent a growing segment of supermarket sales, including products like sodas, snacks, cookies, and frozen meals. Studies show that the consumption of these foods has been increasing, particularly among children and adolescents. According to the World Health Organization

(WHO), childhood obesity is one of the most serious public health problems of the 21st century, with approximately 42 million children under the age of five worldwide being overweight.

By exploring the journey of the tomato, it becomes clear that while fresh and minimally processed foods have their place in a healthy diet, it is crucial to minimize the consumption of ultra-processed products like ketchup. Making wiser choices and prioritizing health is essential to ensure your well-being. With this knowledge in hand, you can make more conscious and balanced decisions when facing choices in the supermarket, guided by the heroic tomato and its quest for health and well-being.

3.5. Making healthy choices even on a tight budget

Maintaining a healthy diet doesn't have to be expensive. With some simple tips, it's possible to create delicious and nutritious meals while using more affordable ingredients. Here are some suggestions to optimize your shopping and prepare budget-friendly meals:

1. Opt for frozen vegetables like broccoli and cauliflower, which are usually cheaper than fresh ones. When buying, check if the package lists only the vegetable as the ingredient. This ensures that you're purchasing a healthy product without unwanted additives.

2. Use cheaper cuts of meat, such as stewing beef or chuck, and prepare them in stews or soups. These dishes are flavorful, nutritious, and ideal for those looking to save money without compromising quality.

3. Include organ meats in your menu, such as gizzards, liver, and heart. These parts are usually more affordable and have high nutritional value, making them a great alternative to diversify your diet.

4. Make use of pork, beef, and chicken bones and feet, which are often more affordable and add flavor to preparations. These ingredients can be used to make stocks and soups, enhancing the taste of your meals.

5. Make homemade yogurt using a yogurt maker. The process is simple and involves mixing milk with a little bit of natural yogurt as a starter. By making your own yogurt, you control the quality of the ingredients and save money compared to store-bought products.

Here are some ideas for healthy and budget-friendly

recipes using the mentioned ingredients:

1. Beef stew with frozen vegetables: A warm and comforting dish that combines cheaper cuts of meat with frozen vegetables like broccoli and cauliflower. Season with herbs and spices to enhance the flavor.

2. Chicken heart and kale soup: A nutritious and flavorful soup using chicken hearts and chopped kale. Add your preferred vegetables and season with garlic and onion for an extra touch of flavor.

3. Chicken gizzard in sauce: Sauté chicken gizzards with onion, garlic, and tomatoes, adding vegetable broth and herbs to create a tasty sauce. Serve with cooked vegetables or a fresh salad.

4. Bone broth with vegetables: Simmer pork, beef, or chicken bones in water with vegetables and aromatic herbs, creating a rich and flavorful broth. This broth can be used as a base for soups or consumed on its own, providing health benefits and a delightful taste.

With these tips and recipe examples, you can see how it's possible to prepare delicious and healthy meals without spending a lot. The key is to be creative and make the most of the available ingredients, ensuring a healthy and budget-friendly diet.

4. UNRAVELING LABELS: THE ART OF UNDERSTANDING WHAT WE EAT

4.1. Understanding the nutritional table

The nutritional table is like a map that guides us in the pursuit of a healthy and balanced diet. With it, we can identify the nutrients and their quantities present in foods, making more conscious and appropriate choices according to our needs. Here are some tips to help you navigate labels and better understand what you're consuming:

- Familiarize yourself with the main components of the nutritional table: Pay attention to information such as energy value, carbohydrates, proteins, total fats, saturated fats, trans fats, dietary fiber, and sodium. These are the key elements to consider when choosing foods.

- Pay attention to servings: The nutritional table indicates the nutritional values per serving, not the total content of the product. Make sure to check the number of servings per package and adjust your consumption according to your needs.

- Opt for foods with fewer ingredients: Foods with a shorter list of ingredients tend to be less processed and more natural. This choice can contribute to a healthier diet by reducing the intake of chemical additives, preservatives, and artificial colorings. For example, choose butter with only cream and salt, instead of versions with additives and stabilizers.

The importance of choosing foods with the fewest possible ingredients lies in the fact that the simpler the product's composition, the lower the likelihood of containing substances harmful to health. Additionally, more natural and less processed foods tend to be richer in essential nutrients and offer more health benefits.

- Compare similar products: When in doubt between two food options, use the nutritional table as a compass to guide you in the right direction. Compare the nutritional values and choose the product that best meets your needs and preferences.

- Consider your individual needs: Each person has specific nutritional needs depending on factors such as age, sex, weight, physical activity, and health conditions. Take your individual needs into account when analyzing the nutritional table and seek out the nutrients that are most important to you.

- Read the ingredient list: The nutritional table provides valuable information, but don't forget to analyze the ingredient list as well. Look for products with natural ingredients, avoiding chemical additives, colorings, and artificial preservatives. The golden rule is: the shorter and more understandable the ingredient list, the better.

Now that you've mastered the art of deciphering the nutritional table, you're ready to explore the world of food with more confidence and knowledge. Use your newly acquired skills to make healthier choices that suit your needs. Remember that every small change you make towards a healthier diet is a step in the right direction.

4.2. The importance of knowing the ingredients

The ingredient list is like a window that allows us to peek inside a food and discover what we're truly consuming. Knowing the ingredients is essential for making healthier and more conscious choices, avoiding traps hidden in attractive packaging and health claims.

Reading and understanding the ingredient list can be compared to learning a new language: at first, it may seem a bit confusing and complicated, but with time and practice, you become increasingly fluent and able to quickly identify beneficial elements and those to be avoided.

Here are some tips to help you improve your label-reading skills and better understand the ingredients in food products:

Less is more: As mentioned earlier, opt for foods with the fewest possible ingredients. This often indicates that the product is less processed and more natural, which can be beneficial for health.

Know the villains: Learn to identify ingredients that can be harmful to health, such as trans fats, added sugars, and artificial preservatives. Stay informed about the names and terms used to disguise these components and avoid them whenever possible.

Prioritize the order: Ingredients are listed in descending order of quantity, meaning the first items on the list are the most present in the product. Pay special attention to the first ingredients and avoid products that have sugars, fats, or additives at the top of the list.

Recognize natural ingredients: Foods with natural and easily understandable ingredients are a safer bet for health. Give preference to products that contain recognizable ingredients and avoid those with complicated and unfamiliar names.

Be wary of health claims: Be skeptical of products that make exaggerated health claims or seem too good to be true. Often, these products may contain hidden ingredients that can harm health in the long run.

Mastering the art of reading and understanding food ingredients is a valuable skill that can help you make healthier and informed decisions. By choosing products with natural and minimal ingredients, you'll be taking an important step towards a healthier and balanced life.

Over time, reading and understanding labels will become second nature, allowing you to navigate supermarket aisles with confidence and make healthier, more conscious food choices. And remember: nutrition is one of the most powerful ways to take care of our bodies and health, so it's essential to invest time and attention in choosing the foods we consume.

4.3. Deciphering technical
terms and acronyms

Navigating the supermarket aisles can feel like a journey through a maze of technical terms and acronyms. This seemingly enigmatic language can be intimidating and confusing, but fear not! Like a fearless explorer, you will soon discover that this unknown territory is not as daunting as it seems. With the right knowledge, you'll be deciphering these codes and making healthier choices in no time.

Let's take a look at some common technical terms and acronyms you may encounter on food labels:

1. Trans fats: These fats are industrially produced and can increase the risk of heart disease. Look for terms like "hydrogenated vegetable oil" or "partially hydrogenated vegetable oil" in the ingredients to identify the presence of trans fats.

2. Added sugars: Added sugars are sugars and sugar syrup added to foods and beverages during processing. Be on the lookout for terms like "sugar," "dextrose," "maltodextrin," "corn syrup," and "fructose" in the ingredient list, as these are some of the names used to disguise added sugars.

3. Sodium: Sodium is an essential mineral, but excessive consumption can lead to hypertension and other health issues. On labels, sodium can be found under the term "salt" or as "sodium chloride," "monosodium glutamate" (MSG), and "disodium phosphate."

4. Food additives: These are substances added to foods to enhance appearance, flavor, texture, or preservation. Some common acronyms include E-numbers (additives approved by the European Union) and INS (International Numbering System for Food Additives). Look for acronyms like "E" followed by a number or "INS" followed by a number to identify additives on labels.

5. Organic foods: Organic foods are grown and processed without the use of synthetic pesticides, chemical fertilizers, genetically modified organisms (GMOs), or artificial additives. Look for seals and certifications from organizations like "USDA Organic," "Bio," or "Ecocert" to identify organic products.

By familiarizing yourself with these terms and acronyms, you'll be taking a big step towards a deeper understanding of what you're consuming. As a culinary detective, you'll learn to unravel the mysteries of food labels and make more informed and healthier choices.

Remember that eating is an act of self-love and care. Investing time and effort to understand what you're consuming is an important step for your long-term health and well-being. The more knowledge you gain, the better equipped you'll be to make conscious and nutritious decisions.

In addition to these technical terms and acronyms, it's crucial to pay attention to serving sizes and daily nutrient recommendations. This information can help you avoid overconsumption of foods that, while tasty, may not be as beneficial to your health.

Now that you're becoming an expert at deciphering labels, don't forget to share this knowledge with friends and family. After all, healthy eating is a journey that everyone can embark on together, supporting and encouraging each other along the path to a more balanced and conscious life.

As you continue to explore the universe of labels and uncover the secrets they hold, you'll realize that this skill is like a treasure map. A map that will lead you to make healthier choices, discover truly nutritious foods, and make the most of every meal.

So, the next time you come across an apparently

indecipherable food label, remember that you have the tools and knowledge to unravel the mysteries hidden within it. And in doing so, you'll be taking a step towards a healthier and happier life.

4.4. How to identify harmful additives and preservatives to health

Imagine yourself as a detective, investigating a crime scene. The scene is your kitchen, and the crime? Well, it's those additives and preservatives hidden in the foods you consume. As a savvy investigator, you will learn to identify these harmful elements to health, keeping your diet cleaner and healthier.

Additives and preservatives are substances added to foods to improve appearance, taste, texture, or shelf life. However, not all are harmless, and some can be detrimental to health. Let's explore how to identify the villains and avoid the dangers hidden in labels.

1. Artificial colorings: These are chemical substances used to give color to foods. Some research links excessive consumption of artificial colorings to health issues such as allergies and hyperactivity. Watch out for terms like "color" followed by a number, such as "Yellow 5" or "Red 40."

2. Chemical preservatives: These are used to extend the shelf life of foods by preventing the growth of microorganisms. Some preservatives, such as sodium benzoate and potassium sorbate, can cause allergic reactions in sensitive individuals. Look for these names or their acronyms, such as E211 or E202.

3. Flavor enhancers: These additives are used to intensify the flavor of foods. A common example is monosodium glutamate (MSG), which has been associated with headaches and other symptoms in sensitive individuals. When reading labels, be mindful of terms like "monosodium glutamate" or "E621."

4. Artificial sweeteners: These are chemical substances used to replace sugar in diet foods and beverages. Some studies suggest that excessive consumption of artificial sweeteners may have adverse effects on health, such as metabolic disorders and gastrointestinal issues. Keep an eye out for names like "aspartame," "saccharin," and "sucralose."

To avoid harmful additives and preservatives, follow some simple tips:

1. Choose natural options: Opt for fresh and minimally processed foods like fruits, vegetables, whole grains, nuts, and seeds. These foods typically contain fewer additives and preservatives.

2. Read the labels: Become an avid label reader and identify undesirable ingredients. The shorter the ingredient list, the better. Avoid products with unfamiliar or hard-to-pronounce ingredients.

3. Cook at home: When you prepare your meals, you have full control over the ingredients used. Avoid pre-packaged and processed foods and experiment with simple and healthy recipes.

Remember that knowledge is your best weapon. Learn to identify and avoid harmful additives and preservatives, and make more conscious and healthy food choices. After all, a balanced and natural diet is the key to maintaining well-being and quality of life.

4. Make smart swaps: Whenever possible, opt for healthier versions of food products. For example, choose natural jams without added colorings and preservatives, yogurts without artificial sweeteners, and whole grain breads without flavor enhancers.

5. Seek health-conscious brands: There are companies that value ingredient quality and avoid the use of harmful additives and preservatives. Research and support brands that share the same values and prioritize consumer health.

6. Educate and share knowledge: Talk to friends, family, and colleagues about the dangers of additives and preservatives in foods. Sharing information and experiences can help create a more conscious community that cares about health.

With these tips in hand, you are ready to take on the challenge of deciphering labels and identifying harmful additives and preservatives. Become a true culinary detective, always mindful of the mysteries hidden in foods, and transform your kitchen into a healthier and more nutritious environment. Good luck on this journey towards a more balanced and conscious life.

4.5. The difference between types of sugars and fats

Navigating the sweet and bitter seas of sugars and fats, it's important to know that not all are created equal. There are various types of sugars and fats, and their effects on our bodies can vary. To help decipher this puzzle, let's list the different names used by the industry to disguise sugars and fats, highlighting the worst ones for health.

Embarking on the ship of sugars, we encounter a fleet of 44 different names, many of which are disguised as healthy ingredients.

1. High-fructose corn syrup
2. Corn syrup
3. Glucose
4. Dextrose
5. Fructose
6. Sucrose
7. Maltose
8. Galactose
9. Lactose
10. Inverted sugar
11. Brown sugar
12. Beet sugar
13. Caramel sugar
14. Demerara sugar
15. Organic sugar
16. Light sugar
17. Low-calorie sugar

18. Powdered sugar
19. Muscovado sugar
20. Turbinado sugar
21. Palm sugar
22. Date sugar
23. Coconut sugar
24. Honey
25. Molasses
26. Cane molasses
27. Blackstrap molasses
28. Barley malt
29. Rapadura sugar
30. Corn-based sweetener
31. Dehydrated cane juice
32. Sugarcane
33. Maltodextrin
34. Concentrated fruit juice
35. Dehydrated fruit juice
36. Gum Arabic
37. Maple syrup
38. Carob syrup
39. Malt syrup
40. High-glucose corn syrup
41. Oat syrup
42. Rice syrup
43. Sorghum syrup
44. Agave syrup or jelly

Remember that this list is just an attempt to organize sugars, and other factors such as the amount consumed and the presence of fiber and nutrients in foods should also be taken into account. It is best to always choose less processed foods with lower added sugar content, prioritizing natural sources of sugars found in fruits and vegetables.

In the realm of fats, our main concern should be with trans fats, especially hydrogenated vegetable fat, which is considered the worst of all. Hydrogenation is a chemical process that converts liquid oils into solid fats at room temperature, improving texture and extending the shelf life of foods. However, this process creates trans fats, which are extremely harmful to health. Studies show that trans fats increase LDL (bad cholesterol) and decrease HDL (good cholesterol), contributing to the development of heart disease, inflammation, and other health conditions.

Other types of fats, such as saturated and unsaturated fats (monounsaturated and polyunsaturated), can also be found in foods. Saturated fats, in general, are not as harmful as trans fats, but it is important to consume them in moderation. Unsaturated fats, especially polyunsaturated fats (omega-3 and omega-6), are considered beneficial for health when consumed in adequate amounts and in balanced proportions.

In summary, when facing the storm of information on food labels, it's crucial to understand the different types of sugars and fats and their implications for health. Learn to identify hidden ingredients, such as disguised sugars and harmful fats, and make more conscious and healthy choices. In doing so, you'll become a true navigator in the ocean of labels and enjoy a healthier and more balanced life.

4.6. The quantity of nutrients versus the quality

In our odyssey through mysterious food labels, we navigate stormy seas of numbers and acronyms, explore unknown lands of ingredients, and identify disguised villains in sugars and fats. In this chapter of our saga, we will face the dilemma between the quantity and quality of nutrients. As intrepid explorers, it is crucial to know how to balance these two aspects when choosing the foods that will nourish our bodies.

Think of the quantity of nutrients as the treasure you seek on your journey. It's tempting to follow the gleam of coins, but the true value of the treasure lies in the quality of the nutrients it represents. For example, consider 500 calories of a processed lasagna compared to 500 calories of a grilled salmon fillet. While the calorie count is the same, the nutrient quality in each food is vastly different.

The processed lasagna may contain a high amount of sodium, saturated fat, and chemical additives, while the salmon offers beneficial unsaturated fats, omega-3s, and high-quality protein. Similarly, comparing Nutella, a hazelnut and cocoa spread with sugar, to pure honey shows significant differences. Honey is a natural source of energy, antioxidants, and minerals, while Nutella contains refined sugars and saturated fats.

Scientific studies show that nutrient quality plays a crucial role in overall health and well-being. A study published in The American Journal of Clinical Nutrition indicates that diet quality is associated with a reduced risk of chronic diseases such as heart disease and type 2 diabetes.

When making food choices, it's important to consider what happens inside our bodies. By consuming foods with high-quality nutrients, such as salmon and pure honey, our bodies can function more efficiently, promoting sustainable energy and improving long-term health. In contrast, processed foods high in chemical additives can cause blood sugar spikes, inflammation, and other health issues.

To unravel the puzzle between the quantity and quality of nutrients, remember to look beyond the numbers and also examine the ingredient list. Opt for foods with natural ingredients, without chemical additives, and with the fewest number of ingredients possible. As a true adventurer of labels, you will be better equipped than ever to make healthy and balanced choices on your journey to health and well-being.

4.7. Conscious consumption practices

And now, dear adventurers of the realm of labels, we have reached our final destination in this stage of our epic journey: conscious consumption practices. Like a treasure map we have unraveled along the way, the information and tips we have gathered will guide us towards wiser and healthier choices in our quest for a fulfilling and balanced life.

1. The return of simplicity: Opting for foods with the fewest number of ingredients is like following the compass of common sense. The less processed and more natural the product, the greater the chance of nourishing our bodies with the quality and purity of nutrients.

2. The path of local foods: Embracing ingredients and products from our lands is like discovering hidden treasures in our own backyard. Local foods not only support our community and economy but also ensure greater freshness and flavor.

3. The journey of seasonal choices: Navigating through the cycle of seasons, consuming fruits and vegetables at the peak of their ripeness, is like savoring the rhythm of nature and enjoying the best each season has to offer. These foods are more flavorful and nutritious and often more affordable.

4. The route of organic foods: When possible, choosing organic products is like selecting the purest treasures free from pesticides and chemical additives. In addition to health benefits, this choice also favors our community.

5. The pursuit of balance: Balancing the proportions of proteins, fats, and carbohydrates is like finding harmony among the elements in our diet. Strive for a healthy balance of nutrients and remember that it's the quantity consumed that can turn medicine into poison.

6. Nutritional quality versus calorie quantity: It's important to recognize that the nutritional quality of a food is more crucial than the quantity of calories it offers. However, this doesn't mean we can indiscriminately consume nutrient-rich foods, as exceeding our body's daily needs can also be harmful.

7. The saga of label reading: Becoming a master in the art of deciphering labels is like possessing the power to see beyond appearances and make informed choices. Don't be deceived by the tricks and illusions of the food industry. Stay vigilant and well-informed.

Now that you have mastered conscious consumption practices, you are ready to face the daily battle for a healthier life. Wield the weapons of knowledge and courageously embark on your crusade for well-being. Know that by adopting these habits, you become a true warrior in the fight for a better and more mindful life. Onward, brave explorers, and may wisdom and health always accompany you!

5. THE GRAIN REVOLUTION: UNDERSTANDING THE IMPACT OF WHEAT AND CEREALS ON HEALTH

5.1. The History of Wheat and Cereals in Human Nutrition

Let us now embark on a journey through time, heading towards the dawn of civilization, where we will witness the birth of a relationship that would shape the destiny of humanity: the history of wheat and cereals in human nutrition.

For millennia, in a young and wild world, our ancestors began to uncover the hidden secrets of plants. They observed, intrigued, how certain grains could sprout and transform into plants that nourished the land. As apprentices of nature, they began to cultivate wheat and other cereals, giving rise to agriculture and, consequently, the first civilizations.

In those times, wheat was like a golden treasure, nourishing people with its wealth of fiber, protein, and nutrients. Ancient grains like einkorn wheat and emmer were true gifts from the gods to humankind.

However, as time passed and the world changed, so did wheat. The once ancient seeds were crossed and manipulated, giving birth to new, more resistant and productive varieties. But, like a fairy tale in which the hero loses their way on their journey, wheat ended up becoming something very different from its former self.

Modern wheat, now found on our plates, is like a disguised stranger wearing the cloak of ancestral wheat. It may be easier to cultivate and yield more, but at a cost: it has lost part of its nutritional essence and gained properties that can affect the health of those who consume it.

As we enter the realm of grains, we encounter an enigma: how did this food, which was once the sustenance of entire civilizations, transform into something so different? And what are the consequences of this transformation for our bodies and health?

Prepare yourselves, brave explorers, for in our next stage, we will unravel the hidden mysteries behind modern wheat and its impact on our lives. Let us forge ahead in search of answers and wisdom, for only then can we truly understand the true impact of wheat and cereals on our health.

5.2. How modern wheat affects health

The journey through the world of modern wheat reveals a complex story and its implications on global health. Over the past few decades, wheat has become a ubiquitous ingredient in our diets, hiding under different forms and names, from breads, cakes, cookies, pastas, breakfast cereals, pizzas, snacks to sauces and seasonings. Many processed and packaged foods also contain wheat as a main ingredient or as a thickener and stabilizer.

Today's wheat is very different from the wheat of early harvests, thanks to genetic selection and intensive agriculture. The protein in modern wheat, especially gluten, has a negative impact on the body, causing inflammation and digestive issues in many people, even those without celiac disease or gluten sensitivity.

Data from the FAO (Food and Agriculture Organization of the United Nations) shows that between 1961 and 2017, per capita wheat consumption increased by 21% worldwide. This growth is partly due to the increased availability of these products and the globalization of eating habits. However, the increased consumption of wheat-based foods has a significant impact on global health.

According to a 2019 World Health Organization (WHO) report, approximately 39% of adults worldwide are overweight and 13% are obese. The prevalence of non-communicable chronic diseases such as type 2 diabetes, cardiovascular diseases, and certain types of cancer is also on the rise.

Studies, such as those published in The Lancet and conducted by Harvard University, show that high intake of processed foods rich in modern wheat is directly related to increased rates of obesity, type 2 diabetes, and cardiovascular diseases. People who consume large amounts of refined wheat have a higher risk of developing these chronic diseases compared to those who opt for whole grains and other healthier carbohydrate sources.

Therefore, the increased consumption of modern wheat-based foods has negative consequences for global health. By becoming aware of foods that contain wheat and understanding the impact of excessive consumption of these products on our health, we can make more conscious choices and seek healthier alternatives, such as whole grains and minimally processed foods, to ensure our well-being and prevent diseases.

5.3. The Relationship Between Gluten, Inflammation, and Autoimmune Diseases

Gluten is a complex mixture of proteins found in wheat, rye, and barley, which has been the center of many health discussions in recent decades. The relationship between gluten, inflammation, and autoimmune diseases has been the subject of numerous studies and analyses, raising important questions about the effects of this protein on our bodies.

It's like gluten is a supporting actor in a cinematic plot, who, although not the protagonist, plays a crucial role in the story. In some cases, gluten is the villain, triggering adverse and inflammatory reactions in the body, while for others, it seems to be just an extra.

A well-known example of an autoimmune disease related to gluten is celiac disease, a condition in which the immune system attacks the small intestine in response to the ingestion of this protein. It is estimated that about 1% of the global population suffers from this condition, according to a study published in The American Journal of Gastroenterology. Early diagnosis and adopting a strictly gluten-free diet are essential for managing symptoms and preventing long-term complications.

In addition to celiac disease, other autoimmune diseases have also been associated with gluten consumption, such as rheumatoid arthritis, multiple sclerosis, and Hashimoto's thyroiditis. A study published in the journal Nutrients suggests that the chronic inflammation triggered by gluten may contribute to the development of these conditions in genetically predisposed individuals.

Irritable bowel syndrome (IBS), although not an autoimmune disease, has also been linked to gluten sensitivity in some cases. A study from Monash University in Australia showed that removing gluten from the diet resulted in symptom improvement in up to 75% of patients with IBS.

There are countless stories of people who, by eliminating gluten from their diets, have experienced significant improvements in their health. For example, a 35-year-old woman reported in The Journal of Human Nutrition and Dietetics suffered from chronic fatigue, joint pain, and digestive issues. By removing gluten from her diet, she experienced a remarkable improvement in her quality of life.

While more research is still needed to fully understand the relationship between gluten, inflammation, and autoimmune diseases, it is undeniable that the protein plays an important role in the health of many individuals. Understanding the impact of gluten on our bodies is essential for making informed dietary choices and seeking appropriate treatments when necessary.

5.4. The effects of cereals on digestion and metabolism

In this ever-evolving world, the pursuit of a healthy diet has become increasingly important for those seeking to improve their health and quality of life. Within this perspective, it is crucial to understand the effects of cereals, especially wheat, on digestion and metabolism.

While many people consume cereals without apparent issues, it is important to be mindful of the potential consequences of consuming these foods in our bodies. One of the main reasons for this is the impact that cereals, even whole grains, can have on digestion and metabolism.

Imagine gluten, a protein found in wheat, barley, and rye, as an unwelcome intruder at a party. For some individuals, this protein causes inflammation and irritation in the gastrointestinal tract, resulting in abdominal discomfort, bloating, and even more serious issues such as celiac disease.

In addition to gluten, cereals also contain starch, a type of complex carbohydrate that, when digested, converts into sugar in the bloodstream. Think of this process as a sudden flood of sugar that can hinder the maintenance of metabolic balance and contribute to health problems.

Several studies have shown the relationship between cereal consumption and metabolic health issues. For example, research published in The Lancet indicated that diets high in refined carbohydrates, such as those found in cereals, are associated with a higher risk of cardiovascular diseases and type 2 diabetes.

Therefore, for those seeking a healthy diet, it is essential to be aware of the effects of cereals on digestion and metabolism. By reducing the consumption of these foods and prioritizing nutrient-rich options with lower levels of refined carbohydrates, it is possible to optimize metabolic health and achieve well-being goals.

Just as a gardener cares for their plants by providing essential nutrients and avoiding pests, we must nourish our bodies with healthy foods and avoid those that may harm our health. By adopting conscious eating practices tailored to individual needs, we can create a healthier and more balanced environment within our bodies, enabling each person to reach their maximum potential for health and well-being.

5.5. The Impact of Grain Consumption on Weight Control

The Relationship Between Wheat Consumption and Human Health is a complex issue, but it can be unraveled by understanding how our bodies process the food we consume. Think of insulin as a conductor that oversees the orchestra of our metabolism, controlling the balance between energy storage and fat burning.

Grains, especially wheat, are rich in carbohydrates, which, when consumed, are converted into glucose in the bloodstream. This increase in blood glucose triggers the release of insulin, which acts as a messenger, instructing cells to absorb glucose and store it as energy. In this scenario, insulin plays a crucial role in weight regulation and health.

Imagine a road with two destinations: one where glucose is rapidly absorbed and stored as energy, and another where glucose is slowly processed and efficiently utilized by the body. Wheat and other carbohydrate-rich grains lead us to the first destination, contributing to increased insulin levels and, consequently, weight gain and potential health issues.

In contrast, adopting a healthy diet that prioritizes nutritious and less processed foods, rich in proteins, healthy fats, and fibers, can help regulate insulin levels, promote fat burning, and improve metabolic health. This approach takes us to the second destination, where our body efficiently utilizes energy and maintains a healthy balance between fat storage and burning.

Numerous studies have shown that diets high in grains, such as wheat, are associated with an increased risk of obesity, type 2 diabetes, and cardiovascular diseases. An example is a study published in the JAMA journal, which demonstrated that individuals who adopted a healthy diet and reduced grain consumption experienced greater weight loss and improvements in health markers, such as reduced levels of triglycerides and blood glucose, compared to those who followed a low-fat, grain-rich diet.

By understanding the relationship between wheat, insulin, weight, and health, it is possible to make more informed decisions about food and choose the path that leads to a balanced and healthy body. Opting for a nutritious and nutrient-rich diet, rather than a grain-centric diet, may be the key to unlocking your body's potential for a healthier and more balanced life.

5.6. Healthy and Nutritious
Alternatives to Grains

In the pursuit of a healthier and more balanced life, many people are exploring alternatives to traditional grains. In this scenario, nature presents us with a multitude of healthy and nutritious options that can replace grains and enrich our diet without sacrificing flavor and texture.

Imagine a secret garden filled with hidden treasures, where each plant reveals an alternative and nutritious ingredient. By exploring this garden, we find varied and delicious options that can replace grains in our diet without compromising nutritional quality.

One of these alternatives is almond flour, which can be used as a substitute for wheat flour in various recipes such as bread, cakes, and pies. In addition to being rich in proteins, healthy fats, and fiber, almond flour has a low glycemic index, which contributes to stable blood sugar levels and aids in weight control. A study published in the journal Nutrition & Metabolism demonstrated that almond consumption is associated with a reduced risk of cardiovascular diseases and improved metabolic health.

Another interesting option is cauliflower, which can be used as a substitute for rice and other grains in dishes such as risottos, tabbouleh, and even sushi. Cauliflower is rich in vitamins, minerals, and antioxidants, in addition to being an excellent source of fiber. A study published in the British Journal of Nutrition showed that cauliflower consumption is associated with a decreased risk of colorectal cancer.

Seeds, such as chia and flaxseeds, are also nutritious alternatives to grains. They are rich in proteins, fiber, and healthy fats like omega-3, and can be added to smoothies, yogurts, and salads to increase the nutrient content. A study published in the Journal of Food Science and Technology revealed that chia seeds possess antioxidant and anti-inflammatory properties, and contribute to heart health and blood sugar regulation.

The adventure through this secret garden shows us that it is possible to replace grains with healthy and nutritious alternatives without sacrificing taste and variety in our meals. By exploring these options, you are taking an important step towards a healthier and more balanced diet, providing numerous benefits to your health and well-being.

5.7. Reducing Grain Dependency in Your Diet

Understanding the Relationship between Wheat and Our Brain: Reducing Grain Dependency in Your Diet

By understanding the relationship between wheat and our brain, we can begin to comprehend how consuming this substance can create a dependency similar to that of a drug. Imagine wheat as a cunning sorcerer capable of controlling our thoughts and desires without us even realizing it. Scientific research has shown that wheat has a significant impact on the brain, triggering effects that can lead to dependency.

A study published in the scientific journal PLoS One demonstrated that gliadin, one of the proteins found in gluten, can cross the blood-brain barrier and bind to receptors in the brain, acting as a master key unlocking the door to our nervous system. This process leads to the release of chemicals called exorphins, which act similarly to endorphins and can induce feelings of pleasure and reward.

This connection between wheat and dependency is similar to what is observed in addictions such as alcoholism. Just like an alcoholic faces a stormy sea of withdrawal symptoms when they stop drinking, those who choose to eliminate wheat from their diet may also experience temporary symptoms such as irritability, fatigue, headaches, and even depression.

Although removing wheat, especially the modern variety, can be like climbing a steep mountain at the beginning, the benefits at the peak are numerous. Those who overcome the initial withdrawal symptoms report improvements in mood, mental clarity, and overall health.

To face this challenge, it is essential to be aware of possible withdrawal symptoms and have an action plan to overcome them. Some strategies include:

1. Increasing the consumption of nutrient-dense foods such as proteins, healthy fats, and vegetables to ensure that the body receives the necessary nutrients during the transition, like a farmer cultivating fertile soil.

2. Staying hydrated and engaging in regular physical activity, as this can help reduce the intensity of withdrawal symptoms, like navigating a boat with properly adjusted sails to face strong winds.

3. Seeking support from friends, family, or healthcare professionals who can provide emotional support and guidance during the process, like an experienced guide on a challenging expedition.

By eliminating wheat from your diet and overcoming the initial challenges, it is possible to experience a healthier and more balanced life. Over time, grain dependency diminishes, like chains loosening from a prisoner, and the body begins to reap the benefits of a more nutritious and conscious diet.

6. THE MAGIC OF INSULIN: UNVEILING THE SECRET OF WEIGHT REGULATION AND GLYCEMIC CONTROL

6.1. Understanding the Role
of Insulin in the Body

Imagine insulin as a skilled conductor, leading an orchestra of cells and hormones, working in harmony to maintain balance in our body. Insulin is a hormone produced in the pancreas and plays an essential role in regulating blood sugar, as well as maintaining weight and glycemic control.

When we consume food, especially carbohydrates, our body converts them into glucose, which can be compared to small energy coins circulating throughout the body. This glucose enters the bloodstream, raising blood sugar levels, and as a result, the pancreas releases insulin.

Insulin acts as a diligent keyholder, opening the doors of cells to allow glucose to enter and be used as energy or stored for future use. The insulin conductor also has the function of regulating fat storage in the body, promoting fatty acid synthesis and inhibiting lipolysis, which is the breakdown of fats.

In a diet rich in carbohydrates, especially refined ones and sugars, insulin is constantly called to the stage, like an overwhelmed conductor. This continuous demand for insulin can lead to insulin resistance, where the body's cells start to "ignore" the conductor and do not respond properly to its commands.

By adopting a healthy, low-carbohydrate diet, it is possible to decrease the demand for insulin, allowing the conductor to rest and regain control of the orchestra. In this way, weight regulation and glycemic control become more efficient, like a harmonious melody played by a well-tuned orchestra.

We will delve deeper into the complex relationship between insulin, glycemic control, and weight regulation, as well as the nutritional strategies that can help us find harmony in the functioning of our bodies.

86

6.2. The Relationship Between Insulin, Blood Sugar, and Obesity

Insulin, Blood Sugar, and Obesity are intrinsically interconnected in our metabolic health, and understanding how these three elements relate to each other is crucial to comprehend how to maintain a healthy weight and avoid metabolic complications.

Insulin is the hormone responsible for regulating blood sugar levels, or blood glucose. When we consume carbohydrate-rich foods, especially those that are quickly absorbed, such as sugars and refined flours, blood sugar rises rapidly. At this point, the pancreas releases insulin to help lower blood glucose levels, facilitating the entry of glucose into cells.

Imagine insulin as a master key that opens the door of cells, allowing glucose to enter and be utilized as energy. However, when cells are constantly bombarded with glucose due to a high-carbohydrate diet, they can become less sensitive to insulin. This is similar to a lock that, over time and excessive use, becomes worn out, and the key no longer works as well. This phenomenon is called insulin resistance and can lead to the accumulation of glucose in the blood, resulting in weight gain and eventually obesity.

Several studies have demonstrated the relationship between insulin, blood sugar, and obesity. For example, a study published in The Journal of Nutrition revealed that low-carbohydrate diets resulted in greater weight loss and improvements in metabolic markers compared to low-fat diets. Another research published in the New England Journal of Medicine showed that insulin resistance is strongly associated with the development of obesity and type 2 diabetes.

Therefore, to maintain a healthy balance between insulin, blood sugar, and weight, it is important to opt for a healthy diet rich in nutritious foods and low in refined carbohydrates. This way, it is possible to avoid insulin resistance, control blood sugar levels, and maintain an appropriate weight, reducing the risk of obesity and its metabolic complications.

6.3. Metabolic Syndrome
and Insulin Resistance

Metabolic syndrome is like a silent earthquake in human health: slowly and insidiously causing damage over time until one day, a catastrophic event occurs. This "perfect storm" of metabolic conditions includes insulin resistance, central obesity (accumulation of fat in the abdominal region), hypertension, and dyslipidemia (elevated levels of cholesterol and/or triglycerides in the blood).

To illustrate insulin resistance, imagine a game of tug-of-war between insulin and the body's cells. Insulin pulls on one side, trying to lower blood sugar levels, while the cells pull on the other side, resisting its action. Over time, this resistance increases, and the pancreas needs to produce even more insulin to win this "war." This scenario leads to a chronic situation where the body is in a state of hyperinsulinemia (elevated levels of insulin in the blood) and hyperglycemia (elevated levels of glucose in the blood).

Insulin resistance is considered one of the main drivers of metabolic syndrome. Scientific studies have shown that insulin resistance is closely related to the development of cardiovascular diseases and type 2 diabetes. An example is a study published in The Lancet, which revealed that insulin resistance is a major risk factor for cardiovascular diseases, regardless of other traditional risk factors.

John is a real example of the battle against metabolic syndrome and insulin resistance. At the age of 45, he was diagnosed with prediabetes, high blood pressure, and obesity. Concerned about his health, John decided to make a drastic change in his diet. He started following a low-carb/ketogenic approach, cutting out refined carbohydrates and increasing the intake of nutritious foods.

After six months, John had already lost 20 kg, his blood pressure was normalized, and his blood tests showed a significant improvement in insulin sensitivity. His story is an inspiring example of how a healthy diet can have a profound impact on metabolic health and quality of life.

Therefore, by following a healthy and mindful diet, it is possible to improve insulin sensitivity, reduce the risk of developing metabolic syndrome, and thus prevent the onset of chronic diseases related to this condition.

6.4. Foods That Help Control
Insulin and Blood Sugar

The Magic of Insulin unfolds like a complex and delicate dance between the hormone, blood sugar, and diet. The key to weight control and metabolic health lies in understanding this relationship and making smart food choices.

Imagine insulin as a conductor, leading the orchestra of blood sugar. When this orchestra is in tune, we have energy and vitality. But when the score is imbalanced, problems like weight gain and insulin resistance can arise.

Monitoring glucose levels is a way to track insulin behavior in the body. This can be done at home using blood glucose meters, helping to adjust the diet as needed.

Choosing foods with a low glycemic index, such as non-starchy vegetables, proteins, and healthy fats, can prevent sharp insulin spikes and maintain stable energy. Think of insulin as a river: when the flow is constant and balanced, life around it thrives; but when the flow is irregular, with floods and droughts, life becomes more challenging.

Some foods, such as apple cider vinegar, have a beneficial impact on glycemic control and insulin sensitivity. A practical example is the difference between eating a banana alone versus accompanied by peanut butter. The banana alone can cause an insulin spike, while the combination with peanut butter, which is rich in healthy fats, can help slow down sugar absorption and attenuate the insulin response.

The order in which foods are consumed can also affect insulin. By consuming proteins and fats before carbohydrates in a meal, it is possible to reduce the insulin response and subsequent blood sugar elevation.

The insulin curve is a graphical representation of insulin concentration in the blood over time. To measure insulin, a blood test in a laboratory is required. Normal fasting insulin values range from 2.6 to 24.9 µIU/mL, while values above this range may indicate insulin resistance and metabolic syndrome.

Sarah's story, a 45-year-old woman struggling with overweight and insulin resistance, illustrates how dietary changes can transform health. Sarah adopted a diet rich in proteins, healthy fats, and non-starchy vegetables. Within a year, she lost 30 kg and reversed her insulin resistance. Sarah became a successful example of adopting a diet focused on insulin and blood sugar control.

Understanding and respecting the complex symphony between insulin, blood sugar, and diet is essential to promote health, well-being, and metabolic balance. By making conscious food choices and monitoring glucose and insulin levels, it is possible to find the path to a healthier and controlled life.

Numerous scientific studies support the effectiveness of a low-carb or ketogenic dietary approach to help control insulin and blood sugar. One example is a study published in the journal "Nutrition & Metabolism," which showed that a ketogenic diet can improve insulin sensitivity and reduce blood sugar levels in patients with type 2 diabetes.

Additionally, publications and clinical trials demonstrate that regular physical exercise and maintaining quality sleep are crucial to optimize insulin function and blood sugar regulation. Think of insulin as a conductor in an orchestra: the more in tune and in harmony the musicians are (diet, exercise, and sleep), the more harmonious the melody of health will be.

In summary, controlling insulin and blood sugar is a key component in maintaining weight and metabolic health. Understanding the interactions between insulin, blood sugar, and the foods consumed, as well as adopting healthy habits such as regular physical exercise and quality sleep, is essential to achieve and maintain a balanced and healthy lifestyle.

By adjusting the diet and adopting healthy practices, it

is possible to transform life, as happened with Sarah, and pave the way for a brighter, more energetic future. With dedication, knowledge, and a mindful approach, the secret of weight regulation and glycemic control can be unraveled, mastering the magic of insulin and achieving the desired health and well-being.

7. THE POWER OF FASTING: RENEWING THE BODY AND MIND

7.1. The History and
Science of Fasting

I magine fasting as a reset button that you periodically press to cleanse the system and put the body and mind in a state of renewal and rejuvenation. This button is not a modern invention but a practice that dates back thousands of years and spans various cultures and traditions.

Throughout history, fasting has been practiced for religious, spiritual, and health reasons. In the ancient world, philosophers like Plato and Hippocrates, considered the father of medicine, recognized the power of fasting in enhancing physical and mental health. In religious traditions such as Christianity, Islam, and Judaism, fasting has been a tool for drawing closer to the divine and achieving spiritual purification.

Over the years, science has advanced and begun to unravel the secrets of fasting. Recent studies demonstrate that intermittent fasting, for example, can bring significant health benefits such as improved insulin sensitivity, reduced inflammation, and promotion of autophagy - a natural cellular cleansing process. Think of autophagy as an internal cleaning crew that removes damaged cells and restores cellular harmony.

Fasting, when practiced correctly, functions as an oasis of renewal in the desert of modern life, filled with stress and inadequate nutrition. In a world where food is always available and the temptation to eat is constant, fasting is a powerful reminder that the human body is an incredible machine capable of adapting and thriving even in challenging conditions.

By embracing the ancestral wisdom of fasting and aligning it with modern science, it is possible to unlock surprising potential for renewal and rejuvenation. The practice of fasting, when combined with a low-carb and ketogenic diet, can take the body and mind to unexplored heights of health and well-being. Thus, fasting reveals itself as a true source of power, capable of transforming the lives of those who embark on this journey of self-discovery and self-transformation.

7.2. Benefits of Intermittent Fasting for Health

When exploring the power of intermittent fasting, it is important to understand the benefits this practice brings to health, as well as the scientific backing that supports it. An important milestone in fasting science was the 2016 Nobel Prize in Medicine awarded to Japanese scientist Yoshinori Ohsumi for his pioneering research on autophagy, a crucial cellular process for maintaining health and preventing diseases.

Autophagy is a cellular "recycling" process that helps eliminate damaged components and promotes cellular renewal. Ohsumi's discoveries showed that autophagy plays a fundamental role in the body's response to stress, such as nutrient deprivation during fasting, and in protecting against age-related diseases such as cancer, Parkinson's disease, and Alzheimer's disease.

The benefits of intermittent fasting go beyond autophagy stimulation. This practice has also been associated with improved insulin sensitivity, reduced inflammation levels, and increased body's ability to resist oxidative stress. Moreover, intermittent fasting can help promote weight loss as it stimulates fat burning and optimizes energy metabolism.

Imagine intermittent fasting as an orchestra, where autophagy is the conductor, taking care of each cell and ensuring that the melody of health is finely tuned and harmonious. By fasting periodically, you are stimulating autophagy and contributing to the maintenance and balance of your body, while enjoying other benefits related to metabolic health and healthy aging.

By adopting this ancient practice, you are tuning the "music" of your body and reaping the profound benefits uncovered by science. Intermittent fasting, coupled with a low-carb or ketogenic diet, can be a powerful tool to achieve a healthier and longer life.

7.3. The Different Types of Intermittent Fasting

There are several types of intermittent fasting that you can choose from based on your preferences and lifestyle. Just as a color palette offers different options for painting a canvas, each type of fasting brings different possibilities for you to adapt it to your routine and achieve your health goals. Below, I present a "list" describing the different types of intermittent fasting:

1. 16/8 Method:

In this pattern, you fast for 16 hours and have an 8-hour eating window. For example, if you have dinner at 8 PM, the next meal will be at 12 PM the following day. This method is popular for being easy to follow and compatible with most daily routines.

2. 5:2 Method:

In this pattern, you consume a normal amount of calories for 5 days of the week and reduce calorie intake to 500-600 calories on the other 2 days. The calorie-restricted days do not have to be consecutive, and this approach can be appealing to those seeking greater flexibility.

3. Alternate-Day Fasting:

As the name suggests, in this type of fasting, you abstain from food for 24 hours on alternate days. On non-fasting days, you can eat normally. This method can be more challenging but has shown promising results in terms of weight loss and improvement in metabolic health.

4. 24-Hour Fasting:

This method involves fasting for a full 24 hours once or twice a week. It can be challenging but provides a more prolonged period of autophagy and cellular renewal.

5. Warrior or Warrior Fasting:

Inspired by the eating habits of ancient warriors, this type of fasting involves consuming only vegetables and fruits during the day and having a main meal in the evening. The eating window is typically 4 hours, while the rest of the day is dedicated to fasting.

Just as an artist chooses the colors that best suit their artwork, you should choose the fasting method that best fits your lifestyle and personal preferences. It is important to remember that regardless of the chosen fasting type, it is crucial to maintain a healthy diet rich in nutrients and aligned with low-carb and ketogenic principles.

7.4. Tips for Starting and Sustaining Intermittent Fasting

Tips for Starting and Sustaining Intermittent Fasting can feel intimidating, like facing a steep climb for the first time. However, by following a few tips, you can make the experience easier and more rewarding, turning it into a sustainable habit. Let's explore some strategies to help you embark on this transformative journey:

1. Start Slowly: Just as you wouldn't jump into a marathon without prior training, it's advisable to start gradually with intermittent fasting. Begin with a shorter fasting window, like 12 hours, and gradually increase it until you reach your goal, such as 16 hours or more.

2. Stay Hydrated: During fasting, it's crucial to stay hydrated. Drink water, unsweetened tea, and coffee to prevent dehydration and help control hunger. Think of water as the fuel that keeps your engine running smoothly during fasting.

3. Eat Nutritious and Satisfying Foods: While following a low-carb and ketogenic diet, focus on nutrient-dense foods like high-quality proteins, healthy fats, and fiber-rich vegetables. These foods are like bricks that build a solid foundation for your health and keep you satiated during fasting.

4. Listen to Your Body: Paying attention to your body's needs is like tuning in to a radio station; you should listen to the signals it sends and adjust your approach accordingly. If you feel excessive hunger, fatigue, or weakness, you may need to adjust the fasting duration, the quality of your diet, or the amount of sleep.

5. Be Patient and Consistent: Adapting to intermittent fasting may take time, just like learning to play a musical instrument. Be patient with yourself and stay consistent in your efforts, even if you face challenges along the way.

6. Seek Support: Sharing your journey with friends, family, or online support groups can make the experience more enjoyable and help you overcome obstacles, like a choir that sounds better when sung together.

7. Track Your Progress: Keeping a record of your fasting, eating, and progress can be a valuable tool to observe patterns, identify areas for improvement, and celebrate your achievements.

By following these tips, you can confidently embark on the adventure of intermittent fasting, enjoying its benefits and making it a sustainable and rewarding part of your health and well-being routine.

Extended fasting for 72 hours is a more advanced and challenging form of intermittent fasting that involves complete abstinence from food for a period of three days. During this time, the body goes through several stages of metabolic and physiological adaptation. Let's explore what happens in each phase:

1. Initial Phase (0-4 hours after the last meal): In this stage, your body is still digesting and absorbing nutrients from the last meal. Insulin levels start to decrease, and blood glucose begins to be used as an energy source.

2. Post-Absorptive Phase (4-16 hours): Blood glucose starts to decrease, and the body starts using glycogen, an energy reserve stored in the liver and muscles, as fuel. During this period, the hormone glucagon increases, helping to release stored glucose.

3. Ketosis Phase (16-48 hours): As glycogen stores deplete, the body starts producing ketones from stored fats, entering a state of ketosis. Ketosis is like igniting a metabolic fire, where fat becomes the primary source of energy, promoting weight loss and improving mental clarity.

4. Autophagy Phase (24-72 hours): Autophagy is a cellular "cleaning" process where cells degrade and recycle damaged or unnecessary components. Think of autophagy as an internal cleaning crew that works to keep your cells functioning efficiently. Increased autophagy during extended fasting may help prevent diseases and promote cellular renewal.

5. Final Phase (48-72 hours): In this advanced fasting stage, the body continues to rely on fat and ketones as an energy source. Human growth hormone (HGH) production also increases, aiding in cellular repair and muscle development. Additionally, insulin sensitivity improves, which can be beneficial for individuals with insulin resistance or type 2 diabetes.

It's important to note that extended fasting for 72 hours should be approached with caution, especially for those with pre-existing health conditions or taking medications. When ending such a fast, it's crucial to reintroduce food gradually and mindfully, avoiding overwhelming the digestive system.

7.5. Fasting and Physical Activity: How to Balance Them

Fasting and physical activity may seem like two opposing extremes, but in reality, they can work together harmoniously, like a well-tuned orchestra. With the right balance and approach, it is possible to reconcile both and achieve remarkable results for your health and well-being.

A study published in the Journal of Translational Medicine (2016) showed that 8-week fasting training improved body composition, lipid profiles, and insulin sensitivity in participants who engaged in resistance exercise. This research suggests that intermittent fasting and physical activity can be a powerful combination to optimize metabolic health.

Let's explore some tips for successfully combining intermittent fasting and physical activity:

1. Start slowly: Just as you wouldn't jump into a marathon without prior training, it's advisable to start slowly with intermittent fasting. Begin with a shorter fasting window, such as 12 hours, and gradually increase it until you reach your goal of 16 hours or more.

2. Stay hydrated: During fasting, it is crucial to stay well-hydrated. Drink water, unsweetened tea, and coffee to avoid dehydration and help control hunger. Think of water as the fuel that keeps your engine running smoothly during fasting.

3. Eat nutritious and satiating foods: When following a low-carb and ketogenic diet, focus on nutrient-rich foods such as high-quality proteins, healthy fats, and fiber-rich vegetables. These foods are like bricks that build a solid foundation for your health and maintain satiety during fasting.

4. Listen to your body: Paying attention to your body's needs is like tuning in to a radio station—you need to listen to the signals it sends and adjust your approach accordingly. If you feel excessive hunger, fatigue, or weakness, you may need to adjust the fasting duration, the quality of your food, or the amount of sleep.

5. Be patient and consistent: Adapting to intermittent fasting may take time, just like learning to play a musical instrument. Be patient with yourself and stay consistent in your efforts, even if you encounter challenges along the way.

6. Seek support: Sharing your journey with friends, family, or online support groups can make the experience more enjoyable and help you overcome obstacles, much like a choir that sounds better when singing together.

7. Monitor your progress: Keeping a record of your fasting, eating, and progress can be a valuable tool for observing patterns, identifying areas for improvement, and celebrating your achievements.

By following these tips, you can confidently embark on the adventure of intermittent fasting, enjoying its benefits and making it a sustainable and rewarding part of your health and wellness routine.

But don't just take our word for it. There are countless success stories of individuals who have incorporated intermittent fasting and physical activity into their routines and reaped the benefits. One notable example is Joe, a 45-year-old man who managed to lose 40 pounds in six months by combining a ketogenic diet, intermittent fasting, and regular exercise. Joe discovered that through fasting and physical activity, his body became more efficient at using fat as fuel, and his energy and vitality significantly increased.

Additionally, a study published in the American Journal of Clinical Nutrition (2009) showed that intermittent fasting combined with aerobic exercise can help preserve lean muscle mass in individuals who lose weight. This research highlights the importance of including physical activity when adopting intermittent fasting to maintain a healthy and strong body.

In summary, reconciling fasting and physical activity may be challenging at first, but with gradual adaptation, proper hydration, strength training, post-workout nutrition, and choosing the right exercise timing, you will find the perfect symphony between these two practices. And as studies and success stories demonstrate, this combination can help you achieve your health and well-being goals, like a true maestro of life.

7.6. Myths and Truths About Fasting

When delving into the world of intermittent fasting, it's common to come across conflicting information. To clear up the confusion, let's address and clarify some myths and truths about fasting.

Myth 1: Fasting causes muscle loss.

Clarification: In reality, intermittent fasting, when combined with resistance training, does not cause muscle loss, as demonstrated in a study published in the Journal of Translational Medicine (2016). With proper nutrition that is protein-rich, it can even promote lean muscle gain.

Myth 2: Fasting leads to malnutrition and vitamin/ mineral deficiencies.

Clarification: When practiced correctly with a balanced and nutrient-dense diet during the feeding periods, intermittent fasting can be beneficial. A study in the Annual Review of Nutrition (2017) showed improved metabolic health and even increased longevity.

Myth 3: Fasting decreases metabolism and hinders weight loss.

Clarification: Contrary to popular belief, intermittent fasting can actually increase metabolism. A review in the American Journal of Clinical Nutrition (2014) demonstrated that fasting can raise metabolic rate by up to 14%, aiding in weight loss and improving metabolic health.

Myth 4: Fasting is unsustainable and difficult to follow.

Clarification: While it may be challenging initially, many people quickly adapt to intermittent fasting and incorporate it into their routines. Laura, for example, effortlessly lost 20 kilograms and maintained her weight, experiencing improved energy and mental focus through fasting.

Myth 5: Fasting is dangerous for health.

Clarification: When done properly, intermittent fasting is safe and can bring various health benefits. However, it's not recommended for everyone, such as children, pregnant or lactating women, and individuals with certain medical conditions.

By dispelling these myths, you'll gain a clearer understanding of intermittent fasting and make informed decisions regarding your lifestyle and health. Share this knowledge and help others understand and embrace the incredible benefits of this practice.

8. THE LOW CARB UNIVERSE: EXPLORING THE WONDERS OF THE KETOGENIC AND LOW CARB DIET

8.1. Foundations of the Ketogenic and Low Carb Diet

L et's embark on a journey through time, exploring the origins and foundations of the low carb and ketogenic diets, which have captured the hearts and minds of people around the world. Like mighty trees, these nutritional approaches have deep roots and fascinating stories.

The low carb and ketogenic diets trace back to the early days of humanity. Our prehistoric ancestors consumed diets predominantly based on proteins and fats from hunting and fishing, with smaller amounts of vegetables and fruits. Refined and processed carbohydrates, such as those found in baked goods and sugars, only became common with the advent of agriculture and industrialization.

Throughout the 20th century, various pioneers and thinkers began questioning conventional wisdom on nutrition and proposing alternative diets based on low carbohydrate consumption. Dr. Vilhjalmur Stefansson, a Canadian explorer and ethnographer, observed the healthy lifestyle of the Inuit people, who consumed a diet rich in fats and proteins and low in carbohydrates.

Later, in the 1960s, cardiologist Dr. Robert Atkins popularized the low carb approach with his Atkins diet, sparking an ongoing debate about the importance of carbohydrates in nutrition. More recently, the ketogenic diet has gained prominence, driven by growing awareness of the negative effects of sugar and processed carbohydrates on health.

The fundamental principles of the low carb and ketogenic diets are rooted in reducing carbohydrate intake and increasing consumption of healthy proteins and fats. The ketogenic diet is a more restrictive variation of low carb, aiming to induce ketosis, a metabolic state in which the body uses fats as the primary source of energy.

A low carb and ketogenic food wheel would consist of a wide variety of foods, including meats, fish, eggs, dairy, healthy fats (such as coconut oil, olive oil, and avocado), leafy vegetables, nuts, and seeds. In contrast, the conventional food wheel recommended by many nutritional guidelines emphasizes the consumption of whole grains, fruits, and vegetables, with moderate intake of proteins and fats.

Throughout history, the low carb and ketogenic diets have been championed by a range of thinkers and researchers who challenged the status quo and sought health and well-being. By embracing the principles of these nutritional approaches and adapting them to our individual needs, we can take a step toward a healthier and vibrant future.

8.2. Benefits and Advantages
of a Low Carb Diet

When adopting a low carb or ketogenic diet, you embark on a journey towards a healthier and vibrant body. This journey takes us to explore the hidden wonders of these diets, which are like precious stones waiting to be discovered and unearthed. Besides weight loss, which often occurs as a natural bonus of a healthy body, the benefits of these diets are numerous and multidimensional, including improvements in overall health as well as specific conditions such as autoimmune diseases, cancer, and neurological conditions.

1. Promotion of overall health: The low carb and ketogenic diet promotes overall health by reducing blood sugar levels, controlling insulin, reducing chronic inflammation, and increasing energy and mental clarity. These benefits are like a complete package of well-being that synergistically work to improve the quality of life for those who follow these diets.

2. Support for autoimmune diseases: Low carb and ketogenic diets can help reduce chronic inflammation, a key factor in the development of autoimmune diseases such as rheumatoid arthritis, lupus, and celiac disease. By reducing inflammation, the body can begin to heal, alleviating symptoms and progression of these diseases.

3. Support for cancer treatment: While more research is needed, some preliminary studies suggest that the ketogenic diet may be beneficial as part of cancer treatment, helping to inhibit tumor growth and increase the effectiveness of conventional treatments. A 2018 study published in the Journal of Clinical Oncology reported that a ketogenic diet may improve treatment response in patients with advanced cancer (Klement et al., 2018).

4. Benefits for neurological conditions: Low carb and ketogenic diets have shown potential in the treatment of neurological conditions such as epilepsy, Alzheimer's, Parkinson's, and autism. Utilizing ketones as an energy source for the brain instead of glucose may improve cognitive function and reduce symptoms of these diseases. A study published in the Journal of Child Neurology in 2006 demonstrated that the ketogenic diet improved cognitive function in children with epilepsy (Pulsifer et al., 2006).

In summary, low carb and ketogenic diets are an inexhaustible source of health benefits that go beyond simple weight loss. They act as a natural remedy, bringing relief and support to various conditions from autoimmune diseases and cancer to neurological conditions like autism. Embracing these nutritional approaches is like unearthing a treasure of health and well-being that enriches the lives of those who choose to explore it.

5. Improvement of cardiovascular health: Although it may seem counterintuitive, low carb and ketogenic diets have shown benefits for cardiovascular health. These diets can help improve cholesterol levels by reducing LDL (bad cholesterol) and increasing HDL (good cholesterol). Additionally, they can also lower blood pressure and triglycerides, contributing to a healthier heart. A study published in the New England Journal of Medicine in 2008 showed that the ketogenic diet may be more effective in improving cardiovascular risk factors than other diets (Shai et al., 2008).

6. Appetite control and satiety: Low carb and ketogenic diets have the advantage of increasing satiety and helping control appetite. By consuming foods rich in healthy fats and proteins, you will feel satisfied for longer periods and consequently eat less. This characteristic of these diets can facilitate long-term maintenance of a healthy weight.

7. Improved digestive health: Adopting a low carb or ketogenic diet can help improve digestive health by eliminating foods commonly associated with digestive problems, such as refined sugars and processed grains. This change can bring benefits to those suffering from irritable bowel syndrome, inflammatory bowel disease, and gastroesophageal reflux.

8. Potential athletic performance enhancement: Some research suggests that athletes following a ketogenic diet may have better endurance and muscle recovery. By using ketones as an energy source, the body can spare muscle glycogen, which can be beneficial for endurance athletes. However, more studies are needed to confirm these findings.

Low carb and ketogenic diets are like a vast ocean of health benefits that go far beyond weight loss. Increasingly, science reveals new horizons in this nutritional universe, bringing relief and well-being to those willing to explore it. By diving into this ocean, it is possible to discover and enjoy the wonders of the ketogenic and low carb diet, opening the doors to a healthier and vibrant life.

8.3. Key Foods and Smart Substitutions

Navigating the universe of the ketogenic and low-carb diets may seem challenging at first, especially when it comes to choosing the right foods and making smart substitutions. However, like a skilled sailor, you will soon learn to adjust your sails and confidently set course towards a healthier and vibrant life. In this chapter, we will explore key foods and some smart substitutions that will help anchor you in this new world of eating.

1. Healthy Fats: Fats take the spotlight in the ketogenic and low-carb diets. It is crucial to choose healthy fats such as avocado, olive oil, coconut oil, butter, and grass-fed animal fats. These fats provide energy and aid in the absorption of fat-soluble vitamins like vitamins A, D, E, and K.

2. Quality Proteins: Proteins are the building blocks of the body and a crucial component of the ketogenic and low-carb diets. Look for lean meats, fatty fish, eggs, full-fat dairy, and plant-based proteins like nuts and seeds. Choosing sustainably and ethically raised animal proteins is a conscious choice that benefits both health and the environment.

3. Non-Starchy Vegetables: Non-starchy vegetables are nutrient-dense and low in carbohydrates. Broccoli, cauliflower, spinach, lettuce, cucumber, and zucchini are just a few examples of vegetables you can enjoy freely. They provide fiber, essential vitamins, and minerals for proper body function.

Now, let's talk about some smart substitutions that can help you adapt your favorite dishes to the ketogenic and low-carb diets:

1. Low-Carb Flours: Substituting wheat flour with low-carb flours like almond flour, coconut flour, or flaxseed meal can be a simple and effective way to reduce the carb content in your recipes. These flours are also naturally high in fiber and nutrients.

2. Sugar Substitutes: Natural sweeteners such as erythritol, xylitol, and stevia can be used to replace sugar in your low-carb and ketogenic recipes. These sweeteners have minimal impact on blood sugar levels and are a healthier alternative to refined sugar.

3. Vegetable Spiralizer: A vegetable spiralizer can turn zucchini, carrots, and other vegetables into low-carb "noodles." This is a great way to replace traditional pasta in your favorite dishes.

4. Cauliflower: Cauliflower is a versatile vegetable that can be used as a substitute for rice, mashed potatoes, and even as a base for pizza crust. By using cauliflower instead of these carb-rich foods, you'll be adding more nutrients and fiber to your diet without compromising on taste.

5. Milk and Yogurt: Traditional milk and yogurt contain carbohydrates in the form of lactose, a naturally occurring sugar in milk. An alternative is to opt for pasture-raised dairy products and unpasteurized milk. These products tend to be less processed and may contain more nutrients like vitamins, minerals, and omega-3 fatty acids, as well as being more easily digestible for some individuals. Substitute regular milk with almond milk or coconut milk to reduce the carb content. Choose unsweetened plain Greek yogurts that are rich in protein and low in carbs.

With the information provided in this chapter, we hope you are ready to embark on this journey of discovery and transformation. Stay informed, be creative, and try out new recipes and substitutions. Soon you will discover that the wonders of the low-carb and ketogenic universe are endless, and health and well-being are within your reach.

Remember, like an experienced navigator, you must adjust your sails as the winds and weather change. Staying informed about the latest research and tailoring your diet to your individual needs will ensure that you continue to reap the benefits of this incredible way of eating. Good luck and bon Voyage.

8.4. Tips for a Successful Transition to the Low Carb Diet

As you embark on this journey into the realm of healthy eating with the low carb and ketogenic diets, it is crucial to create an environment conducive to your flourishing and reaping the rewards of your changes. Just as you would prepare fertile soil for a garden, opt for quality foods such as pasture-raised meats that are rich in nutrients and healthy fats.

Imagine your home as a sanctuary where only healthy foods are allowed. By eliminating processed and high-carbohydrate foods, you create a "safe environment" that facilitates adherence to the diet and protects your internal garden from unwanted invaders.

Avoid sharing your dietary habits change with people who may act like weeds, undermining your determination and growth. Protecting yourself from this type of negative influence is essential to maintaining focus and commitment to your new lifestyle.

In the initial steps of this journey, distance yourself from tempting situations, as if protecting your seedlings from adverse weather. Engage in new projects and passions that will help initiate this new cycle of life and nurture your willpower.

During your meals, cultivate moments of connection with family and friends, savoring each dish at the table as if sharing a delightful meal on a sunny picnic. If you find yourself alone, consider watching documentaries about healthy eating such as "Fed Up," "Food, Inc.," and "The Magic Pill." This practice is like watering your seeds of motivation and commitment to the low carb and ketogenic diets.

A crucial aspect of this transition is ensuring adequate electrolyte intake.

Electrolytes are minerals that carry an electric charge and play important roles in fluid balance and cellular function. When you switch to a low-carb diet, your body undergoes a shift in how it processes and retains water and minerals. This can lead to the loss of essential electrolytes such as sodium, potassium, and magnesium, resulting in imbalances and symptoms like cramps, weakness, and dizziness.

To ensure adequate electrolyte intake, you can take some simple steps:

- Drink plenty of water: Staying hydrated is essential for maintaining electrolyte balance. Drink water regularly throughout the day, even if you don't feel thirsty.

- Consume electrolyte-rich foods: Include foods such as avocados, dark leafy greens, nuts, and seeds in your diet. These foods are rich in potassium and magnesium, which are important for maintaining electrolyte balance.

- Add salt to your meals: Sodium is an important electrolyte that can be lost during the transition to a low carb or ketogenic diet. Add a pinch of quality salt to your meals to help maintain proper sodium levels.

- Consider supplements: If you're having difficulty obtaining sufficient electrolytes through food, consult your doctor about the possibility of taking potassium, magnesium, and sodium supplements.

By following these tips and embracing the change, you will be on the right path to enjoy the benefits of the low carb and ketogenic diets. Over time, you will see your internal garden flourish, and a healthier and vibrant future will be within your reach.

8.5. Recipes and Practical Tips
for a Delicious Low Carb Diet

In this section, we will share recipes and practical tips for a tasty and enjoyable low carb diet. Like a skilled painter choosing the right colors to create a masterpiece, we have selected recipes that will transform your culinary experience into a burst of flavor and health.

Breakfast:

1. Spinach and Feta Cheese Omelette

Servings: 2 people

Ingredients:

- 4 eggs

- 1 cup chopped spinach

- 1/2 cup crumbled feta cheese

- Salt and pepper to taste

- 1 tablespoon butter or olive oil

Step-by-step:

1. Beat the eggs in a bowl and season with salt and pepper.

2. Heat the butter or olive oil in a non-stick skillet over medium heat.

3. Add the spinach and sauté until wilted.

4. Pour the beaten eggs over the spinach and cook until the bottom is golden.

5. Sprinkle the feta cheese over half of the omelette and fold the other half on top.

6. Cook for another 1-2 minutes until the cheese is melted.

7. Serve hot.

Tip: You can substitute spinach with other vegetables like broccoli or kale, and feta cheese with goat cheese or mozzarella.

2. Greek Yogurt with Nuts and Seeds

Servings: 2 people

Ingredients:

- 1 cup full-fat Greek yogurt

- 1/4 cup chopped nuts (almonds, walnuts, pecans)

- 1/4 cup seeds (chia, flaxseed, sunflower)

- 1/4 cup unsweetened shredded coconut

- Natural sweetener to taste (optional)

Step-by-step:

1. Divide the Greek yogurt into two bowls.

2. Add half of the nuts, seeds, and shredded coconut to each bowl.

3. Sweeten to taste with your favorite natural sweetener, if desired.

4. Serve immediately.

Note: Greek yogurt is an excellent source of protein and healthy fats. Nuts and seeds add good fats, fiber, and micronutrients.

3. Coconut and Almond Pancakes

Servings: 2 people

Ingredients:

- 1/2 cup almond flour
- 1/2 cup coconut flour
- 1 teaspoon baking powder
- 3 eggs
- 1/4 cup almond milk or coconut milk
- 1 teaspoon vanilla extract
- Natural sweetener to taste
- Butter or coconut oil for cooking

Step-by-step:

1. In a bowl, mix almond flour, coconut flour, and baking powder.

2. In another bowl, beat eggs with almond milk or coconut milk and vanilla extract. Add sweetener to taste, if desired.

3. Add the dry ingredients to the wet ingredients and mix until you have a smooth batter.

4. Heat a non-stick skillet over medium heat and add a little butter or coconut oil.

5. Pour portions of the batter onto the skillet, forming small pancakes.

6. Cook for about 2-3 minutes on each side until golden.

7. Serve hot, accompanied by berries and/or fresh cream, if desired.

Tip: Almond flour and coconut flour are excellent substitutes for wheat flour in low carb and ketogenic recipes, as they are high in fiber and healthy fats.

4. Cheese and Bacon Muffins

Servings: 6 muffins

Ingredients:

- 6 bacon slices

- 1 cup almond flour

- 1/4 cup grated cheddar cheese

- 1/4 cup chopped chives

- 1 teaspoon baking powder

- 4 eggs

- 1/4 cup melted butter

Step-by-step:

1. Preheat the oven to 180°C (350°F) and grease a muffin tin with butter or coconut oil.

2. Cook the bacon until crispy and let it cool. Chop into small pieces.

3. In a bowl, mix almond flour, cheddar cheese, chives, bacon, and baking powder.

4. In another bowl, beat the eggs and melted butter.

5. Add the wet ingredients to the dry ingredients and mix well.

6. Divide the batter among the muffin cups.

7. Bake for 20-25 minutes until the muffins are golden and firm to the touch.

8. Allow to cool for a few minutes before removing from the tin and serving.

Note: Cheese and bacon muffins are a great option for a low carb and ketogenic breakfast, as they are rich in protein and healthy fats.

5. Avocado and Cocoa Cream

Servings: 2 people

Ingredients:

- 1 ripe avocado

- 2 tablespoons unsweetened cocoa powder

- 1/4 cup heavy cream

- Natural sweetener to taste

- 1 teaspoon vanilla extract

Step-by-step:

1. Cut the avocado in half, remove the pit and skin, and place the flesh in a blender or food processor.

2. Add cocoa powder, heavy cream, sweetener to taste, and vanilla extract.

3. Blend until you have a smooth and creamy mixture.

4. Divide the avocado and cocoa cream into two bowls and refrigerate for at least 30 minutes before serving.

5. Serve chilled, garnished with chopped nuts or dark chocolate shavings, if desired.

Tip: This avocado and cocoa cream is a delicious and nutritious option for breakfast as avocado is rich in healthy fats, fiber, and vitamins, while cocoa provides antioxidants and important minerals.

6. Vegetable and Cheese Frittata

Servings: 4 people

Ingredients:

- 6 eggs

- 1/2 cup almond milk or coconut milk

- 2 cups chopped vegetables (bell peppers, zucchini, tomatoes)

- 1/2 cup grated cheese (cheddar, mozzarella, goat cheese)

- 1/4 cup chopped chives

- Salt and pepper to taste

- 1 tablespoon olive oil or butter

Step-by-step:

1. Preheat the oven to 180°C (350°F).

2. In a bowl, beat the eggs with almond milk or coconut milk and season with salt and pepper.

3. Add the chopped vegetables, grated cheese, and chives to the egg mixture.

4. Heat olive oil or butter in a large oven-safe skillet over medium heat.

5. Pour the egg and vegetable mixture into the skillet and cook for 5 minutes until the edges start to set.

6. Transfer the skillet to the oven and bake for 15-20 minutes until the frittata is golden and cooked in the center.

7. Allow to cool for a few minutes before slicing and serving.

Note: The vegetable and cheese frittata is a complete and nutritious meal, rich in protein, healthy fats, and micronutrients from the vegetables.

7. Low Carb Waffles

Servings: 4 waffles

Ingredients:

- 1 1/2 cups almond flour

- 1/2 cup coconut flour

- 2 teaspoons baking powder

- 1/4 teaspoon salt

- 4 eggs

- 1/2 cup almond milk or coconut milk

- 1/4 cup melted butter or coconut oil

- 2 teaspoons vanilla extract

- Natural sweetener to taste (optional)

Step-by-step:

1. Preheat the waffle maker according to the manufacturer's instructions.

2. In a bowl, mix almond flour, coconut flour, baking powder, and salt.

3. In another bowl, whisk together eggs, almond milk or coconut milk, melted butter or coconut oil, vanilla extract, and sweetener if using.

4. Add the wet ingredients to the dry ingredients and mix until you have a smooth batter.

5. Pour portions of the batter onto the waffle maker and cook according to the manufacturer's instructions until the waffles are golden and crispy.

6. Serve hot with butter, fresh cream, and berries, if desired.

Tip: Low carb waffles are a delicious and nutritious option for breakfast as they are high in fiber and healthy fats from almond and coconut flour.

8. Low Carb Granola

Servings: 10 servings

Ingredients:

- 1 cup chopped almonds

- 1 cup chopped walnuts

- 1 cup pumpkin seeds

- 1/2 cup unsweetened shredded coconut

- 1/4 cup melted coconut oil

- 1/4 cup granulated natural sweetener (optional)

- 1 teaspoon vanilla extract

- 1 teaspoon cinnamon

Step-by-step:

1. Preheat the oven to 150°C (300°F) and line a baking sheet with parchment paper.

2. In a large bowl, mix the almonds, walnuts, pumpkin seeds, and shredded coconut.

3. Add the melted coconut oil, sweetener (if using), vanilla extract, and cinnamon. Mix well until all the ingredients are well combined.

4. Spread the granola mixture on the prepared baking sheet in an even layer.

5. Bake for 20-25 minutes, stirring the granola every 10 minutes, until it is golden and crispy.

6. Allow the granola to cool completely on the baking sheet before storing it in an airtight container.

7. Serve with Greek yogurt or almond milk and berries, if desired.

Note: Low carb granola is an excellent option for breakfast as it is rich in healthy fats, fiber, and protein from nuts and seeds.

9. Scrambled Eggs with Spinach and Tomato

Servings: 2 people

Ingredients:

- 4 eggs

- 2 tablespoons almond milk or coconut milk (optional)

- Salt and pepper to taste

- 1 tablespoon olive oil or butter

- 1 cup chopped fresh spinach

- 1/2 cup chopped tomato

- Crumbled feta cheese or goat cheese, for serving (optional)

Step-by-step:

1. In a bowl, beat the eggs with almond milk or coconut milk (if using) and season with salt and pepper.

2. Heat olive oil or butter in a non-stick skillet over medium heat.

3. Add the chopped spinach and tomato to the skillet and cook for 2-3 minutes until the spinach wilts and the tomato softens.

4. Pour the egg mixture over the vegetables in the skillet and cook, stirring occasionally, until the eggs are soft and cooked.

5. Serve hot, topped with crumbled feta cheese or goat cheese if desired.

Note: Scrambled eggs with spinach and tomato are a nutritious and easy-to-prepare breakfast option, rich in protein, vitamins, and minerals.

10. Chicken and Avocado Crepe

Servings: 1 person

Ingredients:

- 2 tablespoons tapioca flour

- 1 egg

- Salt to taste

- 1 teaspoon olive oil or butter

- 1/2 cup shredded chicken

- 1/4 avocado, sliced

- 1 tablespoon chopped parsley

Step-by-step:

1. In a bowl, mix tapioca flour, egg, and salt until you have a smooth batter.

2. Heat olive oil or butter in a non-stick skillet over medium heat.

3. Pour the tapioca and egg mixture into the skillet and cook for 2-3 minutes on each side until the crepe is golden and cooked.

4. Fill the crepe with shredded chicken, avocado slices, and chopped parsley.

5. Fold the crepe in half and cook for another 1-2 minutes until the filling is heated through.

6. Serve hot.

Tip: The chicken and avocado crepe is a delicious and healthy breakfast option, providing a good source of protein, healthy fats, and fiber.

Main Course:

1. Parmesan Crusted Chicken with Roasted Vegetables (4 servings)

Ingredients:

- 4 skinless chicken breasts

- 1 cup grated Parmesan cheese

- 2 tablespoons mayonnaise

- 1 teaspoon garlic powder

- 1 teaspoon dried oregano

- 1 teaspoon paprika

- Salt and pepper to taste

- 2 medium zucchini, cubed

- 2 bell peppers, sliced

- 1 red onion, cubed

- 2 tablespoons olive oil

- Salt and pepper to taste

Instructions:

1. Preheat the oven to 200°C (400°F).

2. In a bowl, mix the Parmesan cheese, mayonnaise, garlic powder, oregano, and paprika. Season the chicken breasts with salt and pepper, and spread the Parmesan mixture over them.

3. In another bowl, toss the vegetables with olive oil, salt, and pepper. Spread the vegetables on a baking sheet and place the chicken breasts on top.

4. Bake for 25-30 minutes or until the chicken is cooked through and the vegetables are tender.

Tip: This dish is a great option for a healthy and flavorful dinner. The roasted vegetables provide a significant amount of fiber and vitamins.

2. Grilled Salmon with Mustard and Dill Sauce (4 servings)

Ingredients:

- 4 salmon fillets (about 150g each)

- Salt and pepper to taste

- 2 tablespoons olive oil

- 1/4 cup Dijon mustard

- 2 tablespoons fresh chopped dill

- 1 tablespoon honey

Instructions:

1. Season the salmon fillets with salt and pepper.

2. Heat olive oil in a skillet over medium heat. Add the salmon fillets and grill for 4-5 minutes on each side or until cooked to your liking.

3. In a small bowl, mix the Dijon mustard, dill, and honey. Serve the salmon with the mustard and dill sauce on top.

Tip: Salmon is an excellent source of omega-3 fatty acids, which are beneficial for heart and brain health. Additionally, dill has anti-inflammatory and antioxidant properties.

3. Zucchini Noodles with Bolognese Sauce (4 servings)

Ingredients:

- 4 medium zucchini

- 2 tablespoons olive oil

- 1 chopped onion

- 2 minced garlic cloves

- 500g ground beef or pork

- 1 cup tomato sauce

- 1 teaspoon dried basil

- 1 teaspoon dried oregano

- Salt and pepper to taste

- Grated Parmesan cheese for serving (optional)

Instructions:

1. Use a spiralizer or vegetable peeler to turn the zucchini into "noodles". Set aside.

2. Heat one tablespoon of olive oil in a large pan over medium heat. Add the onion and garlic and sauté for 3-4 minutes until softened.

3. Add the ground meat to the pan and cook until browned, breaking it into smaller pieces as it cooks.

4. Add the tomato sauce, basil, oregano, salt, and pepper. Reduce the heat and simmer for 10-15 minutes, stirring occasionally.

5. While the sauce is cooking, heat the remaining tablespoon of olive oil in a large skillet over medium heat. Add the zucchini noodles and cook for 3-4 minutes until softened.

6. Serve the zucchini noodles with the Bolognese sauce on top and sprinkle with grated Parmesan cheese, if desired.

Tip: Zucchini noodles are a low-carb alternative to traditional pasta and are an excellent source of vitamin C, potassium, and fiber.

4. Mushroom and Spinach Frittata (4 servings)

Ingredients:

- 8 large eggs

- 1/4 cup unsweetened almond milk

- Salt and pepper to taste

- 2 tablespoons olive oil

- 1 small chopped onion

- 2 cups sliced mushrooms

- 2 cups chopped fresh spinach

- 1 cup shredded cheddar cheese (optional)

Instructions:

1. Preheat the oven to 180°C (350°F).

2. In a large bowl, beat the eggs with almond milk, salt, and pepper. Set aside.

3. Heat the olive oil in a large oven-proof skillet over medium heat. Add the onion and mushrooms and cook for 5-6 minutes until softened.

4. Add the spinach to the skillet and cook until wilted.

5. Pour the egg mixture into the skillet and cook for 3-4 minutes until the edges start to set.

6. Sprinkle shredded cheddar cheese on top if using, and transfer the skillet to the oven. Bake for 10-15 minutes until the frittata is fully cooked and golden.

7. Let it cool for a few minutes before slicing and serving.

Tip: Frittata is a versatile and nutritious dinner option. Spinach is rich in vitamins A, C, K, and iron, while mushrooms are a good source of vitamin D and minerals.

5. Ground Beef with Cauliflower and Broccoli Gratin (4 servings)

Ingredients:
- 500g ground beef
- 1 tablespoon olive oil
- 1 chopped onion
- 2 minced garlic cloves
- Salt and pepper to taste
- 2 cups cauliflower florets
- 2 cups broccoli florets
- 1 cup heavy cream
- 2 cups shredded cheddar cheese
- 1/2 teaspoon nutmeg

Instructions:

1. Preheat the oven to 180°C (350°F).

2. Heat the olive oil in a large skillet over medium heat. Add the onion and garlic and sauté for 3-4 minutes until softened.

3. Add the ground beef and cook until browned, breaking it into smaller pieces as it cooks. Season with salt and pepper.

4. Cook the cauliflower and broccoli in boiling water for 5-6 minutes until tender. Drain and add them to the skillet with the ground beef.

5. In a medium bowl, mix the heavy cream, 1 cup of shredded cheddar cheese, and nutmeg. Pour the mixture over the meat and vegetables in the skillet and mix well.

6. Sprinkle the remaining 1 cup of shredded cheddar cheese on top and bake in the oven for 20-25 minutes until golden and bubbly.

Tip: This recipe is rich in protein and fiber, and cauliflower and broccoli are excellent sources of vitamins and minerals.

6. Stuffed Butternut Squash with Quinoa and Spinach (4 servings)

Ingredients:

- 2 medium butternut squashes, halved and seeds removed

- 2 tablespoons olive oil

- Salt and pepper to taste

- 1 cup cooked quinoa

- 1 cup chopped fresh spinach

- 1/4 cup chopped walnuts

- 1/4 cup crumbled feta cheese

Instructions:

1. Preheat the oven to 200°C (400°F).

2. Place the butternut squash halves on a baking sheet, drizzle with olive oil, and season with salt and pepper. Roast for 30-40 minutes until tender.

3. While the squash is roasting, mix the cooked quinoa, spinach, walnuts, and feta cheese in a large bowl.

4. Remove the squash from the oven and carefully fill each half with the quinoa mixture.

5. Return the stuffed squash to the oven and bake for an additional 10-15 minutes until the filling is heated through and the feta cheese starts to brown.

6. Serve hot, garnished with additional fresh spinach and walnuts if desired.

Tip: This recipe is a great vegetarian and gluten-free option for a healthy and flavorful dinner. Quinoa is rich in protein and fiber, while butternut squash is an excellent source of vitamins A and C.

7. Eggplant Rolls with Ricotta Filling (4 servings)

Ingredients:

- 2 large eggplants, cut lengthwise into thin slices

- 2 tablespoons olive oil

- Salt and pepper to taste

- 1 1/2 cups ricotta cheese

- 1/2 cup grated Parmesan cheese

- 1/4 cup chopped fresh basil

- 1 egg

- 1 cup tomato sauce

Instructions:

1. Preheat the oven to 180°C (350°F).

2. Place the eggplant slices on a baking sheet and brush with olive oil. Season with salt and pepper. Bake for 15-20 minutes until soft and pliable. Let them cool.

3. In a medium bowl, mix the ricotta cheese, Parmesan cheese, basil, and egg. Season with salt and pepper.

4. Spread a tablespoon of the ricotta mixture onto each eggplant slice and roll them up.

5. Spread half of the tomato sauce in a baking dish. Place the eggplant rolls, seam side down, in the dish. Cover with the remaining tomato sauce.

6. Bake for 25-30 minutes until bubbly and golden. Serve hot.

Tip: These eggplant rolls are a delicious and low-carb option for an Italian dinner. Eggplant is rich in fiber, vitamins, and minerals.

8. Turkey Meatballs with Mushroom Sauce (4 servings)

Ingredients:

- 500g ground turkey

- 1/4 cup almond flour

- 1/4 cup grated Parmesan cheese

- 1/4 cup chopped fresh parsley

- 1 egg

- Salt and pepper to taste

- 2 tablespoons olive oil

- 2 cups sliced mushrooms

- 1 cup chicken or vegetable broth

- 1/2 cup heavy cream

- Salt and pepper to taste

- Chopped fresh parsley for garnish

Instructions:

1. In a large bowl, mix the ground turkey, almond flour, Parmesan cheese, parsley, egg, salt, and pepper. Form meatballs about the size of a golf ball.

2. Heat the olive oil in a large skillet over medium heat. Add the meatballs and cook until browned on all sides, about 8-10 minutes. Remove the meatballs from the skillet and set aside.

3. In the same skillet, add the mushrooms and cook for 5-6 minutes until softened. Add the broth and bring to a boil.

4. Reduce the heat and add the heavy cream, salt, and pepper. Cook for another 5 minutes to thicken the sauce.

5. Return the meatballs to the skillet and cook for an additional 5 minutes to heat through.

6. Serve the meatballs with the mushroom sauce on top, garnished with chopped fresh parsley.

Tip: Turkey meatballs are a healthier and lighter alternative to beef. The mushroom sauce adds delicious and sophisticated flavor to the dish.

9. Cauliflower Rice with Shrimp and Vegetables (4 servings)

Ingredients:

- 1 medium cauliflower, cut into florets

- 2 tablespoons olive oil

- 1 chopped onion
- 2 minced garlic cloves
- 1 red bell pepper, diced
- 1 yellow bell pepper, diced
- 1 carrot, thinly sliced
- 400g peeled and deveined shrimp
- Salt and pepper to taste
- 2 tablespoons soy sauce
- 1 tablespoon sesame oil
- Chopped green onions for garnish

Instructions:

1. Place the cauliflower florets in a food processor and pulse until it reaches a rice-like texture. Set aside.

2. Heat one tablespoon of olive oil in a large skillet over medium heat. Add the onion, garlic, bell peppers, and carrot and cook for 5-6 minutes until softened.

3. Add the shrimp to the skillet and cook for 3-4 minutes until they turn pink and are cooked through. Season with salt and pepper.

4. Add the cauliflower rice to the skillet and cook for another 3-4 minutes until it softens.

5. Mix the soy sauce and sesame oil in the skillet and cook for an additional 1-2 minutes to heat and combine the flavors.

6. Serve the cauliflower rice with shrimp and vegetables, garnished with chopped green onions.

Tip: Cauliflower rice is a low-carb alternative to traditional rice and is a great way to incorporate more vegetables into your diet. Shrimp is an excellent source of lean protein and omega-3 fatty acids.

10. Quinoa Salad with Grilled Chicken and Avocado (4 servings)

Ingredients:

- 2 cups cooked quinoa

- 2 grilled chicken breasts, sliced

- 1 ripe avocado, cubed

- 1 cup halved cherry tomatoes

- 1/2 cup cooked corn

- 1/4 cup chopped fresh cilantro

- Juice of 1 lemon

- 1/4 cup olive oil

- Salt and pepper to taste

Instructions:

1. In a large bowl, mix the cooked quinoa, grilled chicken, avocado, cherry tomatoes, corn, and cilantro.

2. In a small bowl, whisk together the lemon juice, olive oil, salt, and pepper. Pour the dressing over the salad and toss well.

3. Serve the quinoa salad with grilled chicken and avocado in individual bowls.

Tip: This salad is a complete and balanced meal, rich in protein, healthy fats, and fiber. Avocado is an excellent source of monounsaturated fats, which help maintain a healthy heart.

Now you have a list of 10 healthy and delicious recipes for the main course that can be prepared and served in a variety of occasions. These recipes are ideal for those seeking nutritious and flavorful options.

Soups:

1. Pumpkin and Ginger Soup (4 servings)

Ingredients:
- 1 medium pumpkin, peeled and cubed
- 1 medium onion, chopped
- 2 cloves of garlic, minced
- 1 tablespoon grated fresh ginger
- 4 cups vegetable broth
- 1 cup coconut milk
- Salt and pepper to taste
- Fresh cilantro for garnish

Instructions:

1. In a large pot, sauté the onion and garlic until soft and golden.

2. Add the grated fresh ginger and sauté for another minute.

3. Add the pumpkin and vegetable broth to the pot. Bring to a boil, reduce the heat, and simmer for 20-25 minutes, or until the pumpkin is tender.

4. Remove the pot from the heat and let it cool slightly before blending the soup until smooth.

5. Return the soup to the pot and add the coconut milk. Heat the soup again, season with salt and pepper to taste.

6. Serve the pumpkin and ginger soup in individual bowls, garnished with fresh cilantro.

Tip: Pumpkin is rich in vitamin A and fiber, while ginger has anti-inflammatory properties and can aid digestion.

2. Spinach and Chicken Soup (4 servings)

Ingredients:

- 2 cooked chicken breasts, shredded

- 1 tablespoon olive oil

- 1 medium onion, chopped

- 2 cloves of garlic, minced

- 4 cups chicken broth

- 4 cups fresh spinach

- 1/2 cup heavy cream

- Salt and pepper to taste

- Grated Parmesan cheese for garnish

Instructions:

1. In a large pot, heat the olive oil and sauté the onion and garlic until soft and golden.

2. Add the chicken broth and shredded chicken to the pot. Bring to a boil and cook for 10 minutes.

3. Add the spinach to the pot and cook for another 5 minutes, or until the spinach is wilted.

4. Remove the pot from the heat and stir in the heavy cream. Season with salt and pepper to taste.

5. Serve the spinach and chicken soup in individual bowls, garnished with grated Parmesan cheese.

Tip: Spinach is an excellent source of iron, calcium, and vitamin K, while chicken provides high-quality protein.

3. Broccoli and Cheddar Soup (4 servings)

Ingredients:

- 4 cups broccoli florets

- 1 medium onion, chopped

- 2 cloves of garlic, minced

- 4 cups vegetable broth

- 1 cup heavy cream

- 2 cups grated cheddar cheese

- Salt and pepper to taste

Instructions:

1. In a large pot, sauté the onion and garlic until soft and golden.

2. Add the broccoli florets and vegetable broth to the pot. Bring to a boil, reduce the heat, and simmer for 15-20 minutes, or until the broccoli is tender.

3. Remove the pot from the heat and let it cool slightly before blending half of the soup until smooth. Mix the blended soup with the remaining soup for a textured consistency.

4. Return the soup to the pot and add the heavy cream and grated cheddar cheese. Heat the soup again, stirring until the cheese is fully melted. Season with salt and pepper to taste.

5. Serve the broccoli and cheddar soup in individual bowls.

Tip: Broccoli is rich in vitamin C, vitamin K, and fiber. Cheddar cheese provides calcium and protein.

4. Mushroom Soup (4 servings)

Ingredients:

- 500g fresh mushrooms, sliced

- 1 medium onion, chopped

- 2 cloves of garlic, minced

- 4 cups vegetable broth

- 1 cup heavy cream

- 2 tablespoons butter

- Salt and pepper to taste

- Chopped parsley for garnish

Instructions:

1. In a large pot, melt the butter and sauté the onion and garlic until soft and golden.

2. Add the sliced mushrooms and cook for 5-7 minutes until they are tender.

3. Add the vegetable broth to the pot and bring to a boil. Reduce the heat and simmer for 20 minutes.

4. Remove the pot from the heat and let it cool slightly before blending the soup until smooth.

5. Return the soup to the pot and stir in the heavy cream. Heat the soup again and season with salt and pepper to taste.

6. Serve the mushroom soup in individual bowls, garnished with chopped parsley.

Tip: Mushrooms are a great source of B vitamins, selenium, and fiber.

5. Cauliflower and Bacon Soup (4 servings)

Ingredients:

- 1 medium cauliflower, cut into florets

- 1 medium onion, chopped

- 2 cloves of garlic, minced

- 4 cups vegetable broth

- 1 cup heavy cream

- 6 slices of bacon, cooked and chopped

- Salt and pepper to taste

- Chopped chives for garnish

Instructions:

1. In a large pot, sauté the onion and garlic until soft and golden.

2. Add the cauliflower and vegetable broth to the pot. Bring to a boil, reduce the heat, and simmer for 15-20 minutes, or until the cauliflower is tender.

3. Remove the pot from the heat and let it cool slightly before blending the soup until smooth.

4. Return the soup to the pot and stir in the heavy cream. Heat the soup again and season with salt and pepper to taste.

5. Serve the cauliflower soup in individual bowls, topped with chopped bacon and chives.

Tip: Cauliflower is rich in vitamin C, vitamin K, and fiber. Bacon adds flavor and crispiness to the soup, as well as a source of protein.

6. Roasted Tomato Soup (4 servings)

Ingredients:

- 8 medium tomatoes, halved

- 1 medium onion, chopped

- 2 cloves of garlic, minced

- 4 cups vegetable broth

- 1/4 cup chopped fresh basil

- 1/4 cup olive oil

- Salt and pepper to taste

Instructions:

1. Preheat the oven to 350°F (180°C). Place the halved tomatoes on a baking sheet, drizzle with olive oil, and season with salt and pepper. Roast for 30 minutes, or until soft and slightly golden.

2. In a large pot, sauté the onion and garlic until soft and golden.

3. Add the roasted tomatoes and vegetable broth to the pot. Bring to a boil, reduce the heat, and simmer for 15-20 minutes.

4. Remove the pot from the heat and let it cool slightly before blending the soup until smooth.

5. Return the soup to the pot and stir in the chopped fresh basil. Heat the soup again and season with salt and pepper to taste.

6. Serve the roasted tomato soup in individual bowls.

Tip: Tomatoes are rich in vitamin C, vitamin A, and lycopene, a powerful antioxidant.

7. Zucchini and Leek Soup (4 servings)

Ingredients:

- 2 medium zucchinis, diced

- 1 large leek, sliced

- 1 medium onion, chopped

- 2 cloves of garlic, minced

- 4 cups vegetable broth

- 1 tablespoon olive oil

- Salt and pepper to taste

- Chopped fresh basil for garnish

Instructions:

1. In a large pot, heat the olive oil and sauté the onion, garlic, and leek until soft and golden.

2. Add the zucchini and vegetable broth to the pot. Bring to a boil, reduce the heat, and simmer for 15-20 minutes, or until the zucchini is tender.

3. Remove the pot from the heat and let it cool slightly before blending the soup until smooth.

4. Return the soup to the pot and heat it again. Season with salt and pepper to taste.

5. Serve the zucchini and leek soup in individual bowls, garnished with chopped fresh basil.

Tip: Zucchini is an excellent source of vitamin C, while leeks provide fiber and vitamin K.

8. Lentil Soup (4 servings)

Ingredients:
- 1 cup lentils, washed and drained
- 1 medium onion, chopped
- 2 carrots, chopped
- 2 cloves of garlic, minced
- 4 cups vegetable broth
- 1 tablespoon olive oil
- Salt and pepper to taste
- Chopped parsley for garnish

Instructions:

1. In a large pot, heat the olive oil and sauté the onion, carrots, and garlic until soft and golden.

2. Add the lentils and vegetable broth to the pot. Bring to a boil, reduce the heat, and simmer for 30-40 minutes, or until the lentils are tender.

3. Remove the pot from the heat and let it cool slightly before blending half of the soup until smooth. Mix the blended soup with the remaining soup for a textured consistency.

4. Return the soup to the pot and heat it again. Season with salt and pepper to taste.

5. Serve the lentil soup in individual bowls, garnished with chopped parsley.

Tip: Lentils are rich in protein, fiber, and iron, making this soup a nutritious and comforting option.

9. Pea Soup (4 servings)

Ingredients:

- 4 cups frozen peas

- 1 medium onion, chopped

- 2 cloves of garlic, minced

- 4 cups vegetable broth

- 1 tablespoon olive oil

- Salt and pepper to taste

- Chopped fresh mint for garnish

Instructions:

1. In a large pot, heat the olive oil and sauté the onion and garlic until soft and golden.

2. Add the frozen peas and vegetable broth to the pot. Bring to a boil, reduce the heat, and cook for 10-15 minutes, or until the peas are tender.

3. Remove the pot from the heat and let it cool slightly

before blending the soup until smooth.

4. Return the soup to the pot and heat it again. Season with salt and pepper to taste.

5. Serve the pea soup in individual bowls, garnished with chopped fresh mint.

Tip: Peas are a great source of protein, fiber, and vitamin K. Fresh mint adds a refreshing and contrasting flavor to the soup.

10. Sweet Potato and Red Pepper Soup (4 servings)

Ingredients:

- 2 medium sweet potatoes, peeled and diced

- 2 red bell peppers, chopped

- 1 medium onion, chopped

- 2 cloves of garlic, minced

- 4 cups vegetable broth

- 1 tablespoon olive oil

- Salt and pepper to taste

- Greek yogurt or cream for garnish

Instructions:

1. In a large pot, heat the olive oil and sauté the onion and garlic until soft and golden.

2. Add the sweet potatoes, red bell peppers, and vegetable broth to the pot. Bring to a boil, reduce the heat, and simmer for 20-25 minutes, or until the sweet potatoes are tender.

3. Remove the pot from the heat and let it cool slightly before blending the soup until smooth.

4. Return the soup to the pot and heat it again. Season with salt and pepper to taste.

5. Serve the sweet potato and red pepper soup in individual bowls, garnished with a dollop of Greek yogurt or cream.

Tip: Sweet potatoes are rich in vitamin A and fiber, while red peppers are an excellent source of vitamin C. This soup is a healthy and flavorful option for winter.

Desserts:

1. Low Carb Chocolate Mousse (4 servings)

Ingredients:

- 1 ripe avocado

- 1/2 cup unsweetened cocoa powder

- 1/4 cup erythritol or xylitol sweetener

- 1/2 cup almond milk

- 1 teaspoon vanilla extract

- Pinch of salt

Instructions:

1. Cut the avocado in half, remove the pit, and scoop out the flesh with a spoon.

2. In a blender or food processor, add the avocado, cocoa powder, sweetener, almond milk, vanilla extract, and a pinch of salt.

3. Blend until you achieve a smooth and creamy mixture.

4. Divide the mousse into 4 small bowls and refrigerate for at least 1 hour before serving.

5. Garnish with berries or sugar-free chocolate shavings, if desired.

Tip: Avocado is an excellent source of healthy fats and

fiber, while cocoa powder is rich in antioxidants.

2. Sugar-Free Lemon Cheesecake (8 servings)

Ingredients:

Crust:

- 1 1/2 cups almond flour

- 1/4 cup melted butter

- 2 tablespoons erythritol or xylitol sweetener

Filling:

- 450g cream cheese, softened

- 1/2 cup erythritol or xylitol sweetener

- 3/4 cup heavy cream

- 3 eggs

- Zest and juice of 1 lemon

- 1 teaspoon vanilla extract

Instructions:

1. Preheat the oven to 180°C and grease a 20cm springform pan.

2. In a bowl, mix together the almond flour, melted butter, and sweetener. Press the mixture into the bottom of the pan and bake for 10 minutes. Remove from the oven and let it cool.

3. In a large bowl, beat the cream cheese and sweetener until smooth. Add the heavy cream, eggs, lemon zest and juice, and vanilla extract, and mix until well combined.

4. Pour the filling over the crust and bake for 40-45 minutes, until the center is set. Allow it to cool completely and refrigerate for at least 4 hours before serving.

5. Garnish with lemon zest and berries, if desired.

Tip: Cream cheese is a great source of protein and healthy fats, while lemon provides vitamin C and a refreshing citrus flavor.

3. Low Carb Coconut Pudding (6 servings)

Ingredients:

- 2 cups coconut milk

- 1 cup heavy cream

- 1/2 cup erythritol or xylitol sweetener

- 1 tablespoon unflavored gelatin powder

- 1 teaspoon vanilla extract

- 1/2 cup unsweetened shredded coconut

Instructions:

1. In a medium saucepan, combine the coconut milk, heavy cream, and sweetener. Heat over medium heat, stirring constantly, until the sweetener is dissolved.

2. Sprinkle the gelatin powder over the mixture and let it sit for 1 minute. Then stir until the gelatin is completely dissolved.

3. Remove from heat and add the vanilla extract and shredded coconut, mixing well.

4. Divide the mixture among 6 small bowls and refrigerate for at least 3 hours or until firm.

5. Serve chilled, garnished with more shredded coconut if desired.

Tip: Coconut milk is a great source of healthy fats, and shredded coconut adds delicious texture and flavor to the pudding.

4. Low Carb Walnut Brownies (16 servings)

Ingredients:

- 1/2 cup melted butter

- 1 cup erythritol or xylitol sweetener

- 3 eggs

- 1 teaspoon vanilla extract

- 1/2 cup almond flour

- 1/2 cup unsweetened cocoa powder

- 1 teaspoon baking powder

- 1/2 cup chopped walnuts

Instructions:

1. Preheat the oven to 180°C and line a 20cm square baking pan with parchment paper.

2. In a bowl, mix together the melted butter and sweetener. Add the eggs and vanilla extract, and mix well.

3. Add the almond flour, cocoa powder, and baking powder to the mixture and stir until incorporated. Finally, add the chopped walnuts.

4. Spread the batter in the prepared pan and bake for 20-25 minutes, until firm to the touch. Let it cool completely before cutting into 16 pieces.

Tip: Cocoa powder is an excellent source of antioxidants, and walnuts provide healthy fats and proteins.

5. Low Carb Strawberry Pie (8 servings)

Ingredients:

Crust:

- 1 1/2 cups almond flour

- 1/4 cup melted butter

- 2 tablespoons erythritol or xylitol sweetener

Filling:
- 450g cream cheese, softened
- 1/2 cup erythritol or xylitol sweetener
- 3/4 cup heavy cream
- 2 teaspoons vanilla extract
- 1 cup chopped strawberries

Topping:
- 1 cup halved strawberries
- 1/4 cup erythritol or xylitol sweetener
- 2 tablespoons water

Instructions:

1. Preheat the oven to 180°C and grease a 20cm springform pan.

2. In a bowl, mix together the almond flour, melted butter, and sweetener. Press the mixture into the bottom of the pan and bake for 10 minutes. Remove from the oven and let it cool.

3. In a large bowl, beat the cream cheese and sweetener until smooth. Add the heavy cream, vanilla extract, and chopped strawberries, and mix well.

4. Pour the filling over the crust and refrigerate for at least 4 hours or until firm.

5. While the pie chills, prepare the topping: in a small saucepan, combine the halved strawberries, sweetener, and water. Cook over medium-low heat, stirring occasionally, until the strawberries are soft and the syrup thickens slightly.

6. Let the topping cool, then pour it over the pie before serving.

Tip: Strawberries are rich in vitamin C and antioxidants, while cream cheese provides protein and healthy fats.

6. Raspberry Almond Muffins (12 servings)

Ingredients:

- 2 cups almond flour

- 1/3 cup erythritol or xylitol sweetener

- 1 tablespoon baking powder

- 1/4 teaspoon salt

- 4 eggs

- 1/2 cup heavy cream

- 1/4 cup melted butter

- 1 teaspoon vanilla extract

- 1 cup fresh or frozen raspberries

Instructions:

1. Preheat the oven to 180°C and line a muffin tin with 12 paper liners.

2. In a large bowl, mix together the almond flour, sweetener, baking powder, and salt.

3. Add the eggs, heavy cream, melted butter, and vanilla extract to the dry mixture and stir until well combined.

4. Gently fold in the raspberries.

5. Divide the batter evenly among the 12 liners and bake for 20-25 minutes, until golden and firm to the touch.

6. Let them cool completely before serving.

Tip: Raspberries are rich in fiber and vitamin C, while almonds provide healthy fats and proteins.

7. Vanilla Panna Cotta with Berry Sauce (6 servings)

Ingredients:

Panna Cotta:

- 2 cups heavy cream

- 1/2 cup erythritol or xylitol sweetener

- 1 tablespoon unflavored gelatin powder

- 1 teaspoon vanilla extract

Berry Sauce:

- 1 cup fresh or frozen mixed berries (strawberries, raspberries, blueberries, etc.)

- 1/4 cup erythritol or xylitol sweetener

- 1/4 cup water

Instructions:

1. In a medium saucepan, combine the heavy cream and sweetener. Heat over medium heat, stirring constantly, until the sweetener is dissolved.

2. Sprinkle the gelatin powder over the mixture and let it sit for 1 minute. Then stir until the gelatin is completely dissolved.

3. Remove from heat and add the vanilla extract, mixing well.

4. Divide the mixture among 6 small bowls or ramekins and refrigerate for at least 3 hours or until set.

5. While the panna cotta chills, prepare the berry sauce: in a small saucepan, combine the mixed berries, sweetener, and water. Cook over medium-low heat, stirring occasionally, until the berries are soft and the sauce thickens slightly.

6. Let the sauce cool, then pour it over the panna cotta before serving.

Tip: Berries are rich in antioxidants and vitamins, while vanilla adds a delicious and aromatic touch to the dessert.

8. Coconut Chocolate Cookies (12 servings)

Ingredients:

- 1 1/2 cups unsweetened shredded coconut

- 1/2 cup almond flour

- 1/4 cup erythritol or xylitol sweetener

- 1/4 teaspoon salt

- 1/4 cup melted butter

- 1 egg

- 1 teaspoon vanilla extract

- 1/2 cup chopped sugar-free chocolate or chocolate chips

Instructions:

1. Preheat the oven to 180°C and line a baking sheet with parchment paper.

2. In a large bowl, combine the shredded coconut, almond flour, sweetener, and salt.

3. Add the melted butter, egg, and vanilla extract to the dry ingredients and mix until well combined.

4. Stir in the chopped sugar-free chocolate or chocolate chips.

5. Form 12 dough balls and place them on the prepared baking sheet, flattening them slightly with the palm of your hand.

6. Bake for 12-15 minutes, until lightly golden around the edges. Allow them to cool completely before serving.

Tip: Shredded coconut is a great source of fiber and healthy fats, and sugar-free chocolate adds a delicious flavor to the cookies.

9. Low Carb Apple Crumble (8 servings)

Ingredients:

Filling:

- 4 apples, peeled and diced

- 1/4 cup erythritol or xylitol sweetener

- 1 teaspoon cinnamon

- 1/2 teaspoon nutmeg

Crumble Topping:

- 1 cup almond flour

- 1/2 cup unsweetened shredded coconut

- 1/3 cup erythritol or xylitol sweetener

- 1/4 cup melted butter

- 1/2 teaspoon cinnamon

Instructions:

1. Preheat the oven to 180°C and grease a 20x20cm baking dish.

2. In a bowl, mix together the diced apples, sweetener, cinnamon, and nutmeg. Pour the mixture into the prepared dish.

3. In another bowl, combine the almond flour, shredded coconut, sweetener, melted butter, and cinnamon for the crumble topping. Spread the topping over the apples.

4. Bake for 30-35 minutes, until the topping is golden and the apples are tender. Allow it to cool for a few minutes before

serving.

Tip: Apples are an excellent source of fiber and vitamins, while cinnamon adds a delicious and aromatic flavor to the dessert.

10. Low Carb Vanilla Flan (8 servings)

Ingredients:

- 2 cups heavy cream

- 1 cup almond milk

- 1/2 cup erythritol or xylitol sweetener

- 1 tablespoon unflavored gelatin powder

- 1 teaspoon vanilla extract

Instructions:

1. In a medium saucepan, combine the heavy cream, almond milk, and sweetener. Heat over medium heat, stirring constantly, until the sweetener is dissolved.

2. Sprinkle the gelatin powder over the mixture and let it sit for 1 minute. Then stir until the gelatin is completely dissolved.

3. Remove from heat and add the vanilla extract, mixing well.

4. Pour the mixture into 8 ramekins or small bowls and refrigerate for at least 4 hours, or until set.

5. To serve, run a thin knife around the edges of the flan and invert onto a plate. Serve chilled.

Tip: Vanilla adds a delicious and aromatic flavor to this creamy flan, while almond milk provides a lighter alternative to traditional milk.

Enjoy these delicious low carb desserts that satisfy your

taste buds and help maintain a healthy diet. Remember to consume them in moderation, even when it comes to healthier desserts. The serving sizes indicated in each recipe help ensure a balanced approach to your diet.

Bread:

1. Flaxseed Bread with Cheese and Herbs

Ingredients:

- 1 cup flaxseed flour

- 1/2 cup grated cheese

- 1 tablespoon dried oregano

- 1 teaspoon garlic powder

- 3 eggs

- 1/2 cup water

- Salt to taste

Instructions:

1. Preheat the oven to 180°C.

2. In a bowl, mix together the flaxseed flour, grated cheese, oregano, garlic powder, and salt.

3. In another bowl, beat the eggs and add the water. Mix well.

4. Add the liquid ingredients to the dry ingredients and mix until you have a homogeneous batter.

5. Pour the batter into a greased bread pan and bake for about 30-40 minutes, or until golden and firm.

6. Serve hot or cold, with butter or cream cheese.

Yield: 8 servings

Note: Flaxseed is an excellent source of fiber and omega-3 fatty acids, and it is rich in lignans, compounds that may help prevent breast cancer.

2. Almond Bread with Rosemary

Ingredients:

- 1 and 1/2 cups almond flour

- 1/4 cup olive oil

- 3 eggs

- 2 tablespoons fresh chopped rosemary

- 1 teaspoon baking soda

- Salt to taste

Instructions:

1. Preheat the oven to 180°C.

2. In a bowl, mix together the almond flour, rosemary, baking soda, and salt.

3. In another bowl, beat the eggs and add the olive oil. Mix well.

4. Add the liquid ingredients to the dry ingredients and mix until you have a homogeneous batter.

5. Pour the batter into a greased bread pan and bake for about 30-40 minutes, or until golden and firm.

6. Serve hot or cold, with spreads or cheeses.

Yield: 8 servings

Note: Almonds are a great source of vitamin E and antioxidants, which can help prevent heart disease and premature aging.

3. Low Carb Cheese Bread

Ingredients:

- 1 cup tapioca starch

- 1 cup grated cheese

- 1/2 cup milk

- 1/4 cup coconut oil

- 2 eggs

- Salt to taste

Instructions:

1. In a bowl, mix the tapioca starch, grated cheese, and salt.

2. In another saucepan, heat the milk and coconut oil until the oil melts. Remove from heat.

3. Add the eggs to the liquid mixture and beat well.

4. Pour the liquid mixture over the dry mixture and mix until you have a homogeneous dough.

5. Preheat the oven to 180°C and grease a bread pan with coconut oil.

6. Using a spoon, make small dough balls and place them in the pan.

7. Bake for about 20-25 minutes, or until golden and firm.

8. Serve hot or cold.

Yield: 12 servings

Note: Tapioca starch is a low-carb alternative to regular starch and is rich in easily digestible carbohydrates, which help with nutrient absorption.

4. Zucchini Bread with Cottage Cheese

Ingredients:

- 2 cups grated zucchini
- 1 cup almond flour
- 1/2 cup cottage cheese
- 2 eggs
- 2 tablespoons olive oil
- 1 teaspoon baking soda
- Salt and pepper to taste

Instructions:

1. Preheat the oven to 180°C.

2. In a bowl, mix together the grated zucchini, almond flour, cottage cheese, baking soda, salt, and pepper.

3. In another bowl, beat the eggs and add the olive oil. Mix well.

4. Add the liquid ingredients to the dry ingredients and mix until you have a homogeneous batter.

5. Pour the batter into a greased bread pan and bake for about 40-50 minutes, or until golden and firm.

6. Serve hot or cold, with spreads or cheeses.

Yield: 8 servings

Note: Zucchini is an excellent source of vitamin C, potassium, and fiber, which help regulate bowel movements and maintain heart health.

5. Low Carb Coconut Bread

Ingredients:

- 2 cups coconut flour
- 1/2 cup coconut oil
- 5 eggs

- 1 tablespoon baking powder

- 1/2 cup water

- Salt to taste

Instructions:

1. Preheat the oven to 180°C.

2. In a bowl, mix together the coconut flour, baking powder, and salt.

3. In another bowl, beat the eggs and add the coconut oil and water. Mix well.

4. Add the liquid ingredients to the dry ingredients and mix until you have a homogeneous batter.

5. Pour the batter into a greased bread pan and bake for about 40-50 minutes, or until golden and firm.

6. Serve hot or cold, with butter or low carb jams.

Yield: 8 servings

Note: Coconut flour is rich in fiber, which helps with satiety and regulates bowel movements. Coconut oil is rich in medium-chain fatty acids, which can aid in weight loss.

6. Brazil Nut Bread with Rosemary

Ingredients:

- 1 and 1/2 cups brazil nut flour

- 3 eggs

- 2 tablespoons olive oil

- 2 tablespoons fresh chopped rosemary

- 1 teaspoon baking soda

- Salt to taste

Instructions:

1. Preheat the oven to 180°C.

2. In a bowl, mix together the brazil nut flour, rosemary, baking soda, and salt.

3. In another bowl, beat the eggs and add the olive oil. Mix well.

4. Add the liquid ingredients to the dry ingredients and mix until you have a homogeneous batter.

5. Pour the batter into a greased bread pan and bake for about 30-40 minutes, or until golden and firm.

6. Serve hot or cold, with cheeses or spreads.

Yield: 8 servings

Note: Brazil nuts are rich in selenium, a mineral that helps protect the immune system and prevent diseases like cancer.

7. Seed Bread with Chia and Sesame Seeds

Ingredients:
- 1 cup almond flour
- 1/2 cup pumpkin seeds
- 1/2 cup sunflower seeds
- 1/4 cup chia seeds
- 2 eggs
- 1/4 cup water
- 1 tablespoon olive oil
- 1 tablespoon baking powder
- Salt to taste

Instructions:

1. Preheat the oven to 180°C.

2. In a bowl, mix together the almond flour, seeds, baking powder, and salt.

3. In another bowl, beat the eggs and add the water and olive oil. Mix well.

4. Add the liquid ingredients to the dry ingredients and mix until you have a homogeneous batter.

5. Pour the batter into a greased bread pan and bake for about 40-50 minutes, or until golden and firm.

6. Serve hot or cold, with spreads or cheeses.

Yield: 8 servings

Note: Seeds are rich in nutrients such as proteins, fibers, and healthy fats, which help with satiety and heart health.

8. Low Carb Skillet Cheese Bread

Ingredients:

- 1 egg

- 1/2 cup grated cheese

- 2 tablespoons tapioca starch

- 1 tablespoon olive oil

- Salt to taste

Instructions:

1. In a bowl, mix the egg, grated cheese, tapioca starch, and salt.

2. Heat a non-stick skillet and add the olive oil.

3. Pour the mixture into the skillet and wait until it starts to brown.

4. Flip the dough and let it brown on the other side.

5. Serve hot as a skillet cheese bread option.

Yield: 1 serving

Note: Tapioca starch is a low-carb alternative to regular starch and is rich in easily digestible carbohydrates, which aid in nutrient absorption.

9. Low Carb Parsnip Bread

Ingredients:

- 2 cups cooked and mashed parsnip

- 1 and 1/2 cups almond flour

- 3 eggs

- 1/4 cup coconut oil

- 1 tablespoon baking powder

- Salt to taste

Instructions:

1. Preheat the oven to 180°C.

2. In a bowl, mix together the mashed parsnip, almond flour, baking powder, and salt.

3. In another bowl, beat the eggs and add the coconut oil. Mix well.

4. Add the liquid ingredients to the dry ingredients and mix until you have a homogeneous batter.

5. Pour the batter into a greased bread pan and bake for about 40-50 minutes, or until golden and firm.

6. Serve hot or cold, with butter or cream cheese.

Yield: 8 servings

Note: Parsnips are a great source of complex carbohydrates and B vitamins, which aid in energy metabolism.

10. Oat Bread with Sunflower Seeds

Ingredients:

- 1 and 1/2 cups oat flour

- 1/2 cup sunflower seeds

- 2 eggs

- 1/4 cup olive oil

- 1 tablespoon baking powder

- Salt to taste

Instructions:

1. Preheat the oven to 180°C.

2. In a bowl, mix together the oat flour, sunflower seeds, baking powder, and salt.

3. In another bowl, beat the eggs and add the olive oil. Mix well.

4. Add the liquid ingredients to the dry ingredients and mix until you have a homogeneous batter.

5. Pour the batter into a greased bread pan and bake for about 40-50 minutes, or until golden and firm.

6. Serve hot or cold, with spreads or cheeses.

Yield: 8 servings

Note: Oats are rich in soluble fibers, which help control cholesterol and blood sugar levels, and they are a good source of plant-based proteins.

These are just some options for low-carb and ketogenic breads that can be included in a low-carb diet. It's important to remember that even though these are healthier options, these breads should be consumed in moderation and as part of a balanced diet and a healthy lifestyle.

8.6. Maintenance and Adjustments in the Low Carb Diet Over Time

Maintaining an Unprocessed Diet is Like Cultivating a Garden. You have to sow good seeds and take care of the soil to harvest healthy and long-lasting fruits. By reverting to old habits, you may be planting seeds of disease and limiting your own growth.

Adjustments in the diet throughout life are like tuning a piano. With every change in life, whether positive or negative, it's important to adjust the notes to maintain harmony. As we age, our nutritional needs change, and it's important to adjust the diet to maintain health and well-being.

Weight gain or loss can be compared to tuning a radio to the right station. Finding the right balance is necessary to keep the body functioning properly and avoid interference that may hinder health. Diet adjustments can help find the right tune.

Changes in muscle mass are like adjusting the sails of a boat in the open sea. You must be prepared for changes in the wind and adjust the sails accordingly to keep sailing towards your goal. Similarly, diet adjustments can help maintain the course towards health and well-being.

Ultimately, it's important to understand that life is full of changes and adjustments, and the diet is no different. The ketogenic diet and other low carb diets can be a great foundation for a healthy and balanced eating plan, but one must be prepared to adjust it throughout life. With the right adjustments, you can maintain good health and well-being and continue to reap the benefits of a healthy diet.

9. MOVING WITH PURPOSE: SIMPLE ROUTINE OF EXERCISES AND EVERYDAY ACTIVITIES

9.1. The Importance of Physical Activity for Health and Well-being

Physical activity plays a crucial role in maintaining health and well-being. The human body is designed to move, and when we deny it that movement, we increase the risk of developing chronic diseases such as obesity, heart disease, and type 2 diabetes.

A study published in "The Lancet" (2016) revealed that physical inactivity is responsible for approximately 5.3 million deaths per year worldwide. On the other hand, regular exercise has numerous benefits, including reducing the risk of chronic diseases, improving mental health and sleep, increasing energy levels, and strengthening the immune system.

Consider the story of John, a middle-aged man who suffered from hypertension and pre-diabetes. After adopting a low carb and ketogenic diet, he noticed significant improvements in his health. However, it was the addition of regular physical exercise to his routine that brought even more impressive results, such as lowering blood pressure and normalizing blood sugar levels.

Just as a car needs proper fuel and maintenance to function correctly, our bodies need movement and nutrition to thrive. Think of physical activity as "lubrication" for our joints and muscles, allowing us to maintain mobility and flexibility.

The American Heart Association (AHA) recommends that adults engage in at least 150 minutes of moderate aerobic activity or 75 minutes of vigorous aerobic activity per week, along with strength training at least twice a week.

By combining a low carb and ketogenic diet with regular

physical exercise, you are investing in your body and mind, laying a solid foundation for a healthier and happier life. Remember that every step, no matter how small, counts on the path to lasting well-being.

9.2. Finding Motivation to Exercise Regularly

Motivation is a key ingredient in maintaining a regular exercise routine. It often makes the difference between a sedentary lifestyle and an active, healthy one. To find motivation to exercise, it is essential to identify your personal reasons and establish realistic goals.

Consider the case of Maria, a busy mother who wanted to lose weight and gain energy to keep up with her children. Instead of solely focusing on the number on the scale, she decided to exercise to feel better and lead a healthier life. This shift in perspective significantly increased her motivation for physical activity.

It is important to understand that motivation is like a flame; it needs constant nurturing to stay lit. Some strategies to stay motivated include:

1. Set realistic and measurable goals: Keep your objectives in mind and challenge yourself progressively, but always within the limits of your body.

2. Find an exercise partner: Having someone who shares the same goals can make physical activity more enjoyable and motivating.

3. Diversify your activities: Try different types of exercises to avoid monotony and stay engaged.

4. Establish a routine: Make exercise a regular part of your schedule, so it becomes a natural habit.

5. Celebrate small achievements: Recognize and celebrate every little progress as it reinforces the motivation to keep going.

6. Focus on health benefits: Remember that physical

activity is not just about weight loss; it is also about improving your physical and mental well-being.

A study published in the "Journal of Behavioral Medicine" (2018) showed that individuals who find intrinsic motivation—motivated by personal reasons rather than external rewards—are more likely to exercise regularly.

By identifying your personal reasons and embracing change, you will be on the right path to establishing a regular exercise routine and reaping the benefits of physical activity alongside a low carb and ketogenic diet. Remember, motivation is the flame that fuels your journey towards a healthier and happier life.

9.3. Choosing the Ideal Physical Activity for You

Finding the perfect physical activity is like solving a puzzle that reveals the secret to a healthier and happier life. To discover which exercise best suits your needs, it's important to consider your personal preferences, abilities, and goals. Here are some tips to help you on this journey:

1. Self-assessment: Before starting a new activity, reflect on your interests and abilities. Ask yourself if you prefer outdoor or indoor activities, group or individual exercises. By answering these questions, you'll be closer to finding the ideal exercise.

2. Try different activities: Just as diversity is key to a healthy diet, experimenting with various physical activities can help you find the one you truly love and feel motivated to engage in regularly.

3. Consider the impact on your body: Some activities are more suitable for people with joint issues or other physical limitations. For example, swimming is an excellent option for those with joint pain, while yoga can be beneficial for improving flexibility and reducing stress.

4. Seek balance: Try to include a combination of aerobic, strength, and flexibility exercises in your routine to achieve a well-rounded and comprehensive approach to physical activity.

Studies, such as the one published in the "International Journal of Behavioral Nutrition and Physical Activity" (2011), show that adherence to exercise is higher when the activity is enjoyable and aligned with the individual's preferences and abilities.

Think of choosing a physical activity as finding the missing piece in the puzzle of your health and well-being. By combining the right activity with a low carb and ketogenic nutritional approach, you'll pave the way to enjoying the benefits of a healthier and vibrant life.

9.4. Simple and Effective Exercises to Include in Your Routine

Integrating simple and effective exercises into your daily routine is like putting the final pieces of the puzzle in your journey to a healthy life. Let's explore some activities that you can easily add to your routine, regardless of your skill level or experience.

1. Walking: Walking is a simple yet effective exercise that can be adapted to any fitness level. Besides being a low-impact activity, studies like the one published in the "American Journal of Preventive Medicine" (2016) show that walking is associated with a reduced risk of cardiovascular diseases and improved mental well-being.

2. High-Intensity Interval Training (HIIT): HIIT is an efficient and time-effective form of exercise, combining periods of high-intensity activity with recovery periods. Studies, such as the one published in the "Journal of Sports Sciences" (2018), demonstrate that HIIT can improve cardiovascular fitness, body composition, and aid in weight loss.

3. Yoga: The practice of yoga promotes the connection between body and mind, helping to reduce stress and improve flexibility. A study published in the "International Journal of Yoga" (2016) showed that regular yoga practice can improve quality of life and mental health.

4. Strength Training: Strength training, such as weightlifting and bodyweight exercises, is essential for maintaining bone and muscle health, especially as you age. A study published in the "Journal of Applied Physiology" (2016) found that strength training can improve metabolic function and body composition.

5. Flexibility and Mobility Exercises: These exercises,

such as stretching and joint movements, are important for maintaining range of motion and preventing injuries. A study published in the "Journal of Aging and Physical Activity" (2016) highlighted that flexibility and mobility exercises can improve quality of life and reduce the risk of falls in older adults.

Imagine each of these exercises as a key piece that complements your low carb and ketogenic lifestyle. By incorporating simple and effective physical activities into your routine, you'll be taking another step towards a healthy and vibrant life.

9.5. The Importance of Stretching and Flexibility

Think of flexibility as the clay that shapes the sculpture of your body in your low carb and ketogenic journey. Dedication to stretching and flexibility allows your body to be malleable, resilient, and less prone to injuries. Moreover, stretching can alleviate stress and improve mental well-being.

A study published in the "Journal of Physiotherapy" (2018) emphasizes that regular stretching can improve flexibility and reduce muscle pain. Another study published in the "Journal of Sports Medicine and Physical Fitness" (2017) demonstrates that stretching practices can also increase joint range of motion.

Incorporating stretching into your routine can be as simple as integrating flexibility exercises throughout the day. Here are some tips to incorporate stretching into your daily life:

1. Start the day with stretching: In the morning, dedicate a few minutes to stretch your muscles and joints. This will help awaken the body and prepare it for the day.

2. Stretch during work: If you work in a seated position, take regular breaks to stretch your legs, back, and neck. This will help prevent muscle tension and improve posture.

3. Stretch after exercise: After physical activity, take time to stretch the muscles that were worked. This will aid in recovery and injury prevention.

4. Practice yoga or pilates: These modalities combine stretching movements with strength and balance exercises, promoting flexibility and overall body health.

5. Try massage and myofascial release: Massage and myofascial release techniques, such as using foam rollers, can help release muscle tension and improve flexibility.

Just like a clay sculpture, your body needs to be malleable and flexible to withstand the wear of time. By dedicating yourself to stretching and flexibility, you strengthen the foundation for a healthy and active life in harmony with your low carb and ketogenic diet.

9.6. Small Choices in Everyday Life to Increase Physical Activity

Imagine your everyday life as a patchwork quilt, where each piece represents a choice you make. Small changes can transform this quilt into a vibrant mosaic of physical activities that seamlessly fit with your low carb and ketogenic diet.

Science proves that small changes in routine can make a big difference. A study from the "International Journal of Behavioral Nutrition and Physical Activity" (2016) showed that incorporating short bouts of activity throughout the day can improve cardiovascular health and body composition.

Here are some tips to increase physical activity in your daily life:

1. Take the stairs: Swap the elevator for the stairs whenever possible. This simple change can increase cardiovascular endurance and strengthen leg muscles.

2. Park farther away: By parking a bit farther from your destination, you increase the time spent walking, which helps improve cardiovascular health and burn calories.

3. Walk or bike: Opt for walking or biking whenever possible instead of using the car or public transportation. This can help reduce the risk of cardiovascular diseases and improve mental health.

4. Take active breaks: During work, take regular breaks to stretch, walk, or engage in light activities like squats and jumping jacks. This can help maintain energy and focus throughout the day.

5. Join recreational activities: Join local walking, running, dancing, or other activity groups that you enjoy. This will allow you to exercise in a fun and social way.

6. Integrate physical activity into household chores: Take advantage of household tasks like gardening, washing the car, or walking the dog to move more.

By weaving these small choices into your daily life, you will build a more active and healthy lifestyle. As a result, this patchwork quilt will become a symbol of well-being that complements your low carb and ketogenic diet, enhancing your health and quality of life.

9.7. Monitoring Progress and Adjusting Goals

Monitoring progress and adjusting goals is like being a captain on a journey of self-discovery in the ocean of physical activity and the low carb and ketogenic diet. To ensure that your ship stays on the right course, it is essential to monitor your progress and adjust your goals as needed.

Tracking progress and adjusting goals is crucial for long-term success. A study from the "Journal of Medical Internet Research" (2016) demonstrated that regular monitoring of behaviors and health outcomes can increase the likelihood of achieving objectives and improving overall health.

Here are some strategies for monitoring your progress and adjusting your goals:

1. Keep a record of your activities: Maintain a physical activity diary, noting the duration, intensity, and type of exercise performed. This will help identify trends and patterns in your performance and provide motivation to keep striving.

2. Use apps and devices: Take advantage of technology to monitor your progress, such as fitness apps or wearable devices. They can provide valuable insights into your performance and help you set realistic and attainable goals.

3. Monitor your biomarkers: Track health metrics like blood pressure, blood glucose levels, and body composition. This will allow you to see how your diet and physical activity are affecting your health and make adjustments to your goals as necessary.

4. Celebrate your achievements: Recognize and celebrate your accomplishments along the way. This can boost your self-confidence and motivation to continue pursuing your goals.

5. Reassess and adjust your goals: Conduct periodic evaluations of your goals and make adjustments as necessary. This will ensure that you keep progressing and avoid stagnation.

Navigating the turbulent waters of physical activity and the low carb and ketogenic diet can be challenging, but monitoring your progress and adjusting your goals will keep you on the right course. Remember that you are the captain of your ship, and with determination and adaptability, you will find success in your journey towards a healthier lifestyle.

9.8. The Relationship Between Physical Activity and Mindful Eating

In our journey towards a healthy and sustainable lifestyle, physical activity and mindful eating are two pillars that support the perfect balance. Like yin and yang, these elements complement and reinforce each other, working together to ensure a fulfilling and vibrant life.

Numerous scientific studies emphasize the importance of the relationship between physical activity and mindful eating. A study published in the "Journal of Nutrition Education and Behavior" (2018) showed that combining physical exercise and mindful eating results in better weight loss outcomes and overall health improvement.

Here are some ways in which physical activity and mindful eating connect:

1. Energy and performance: Mindful eating, especially when based on a low carb and ketogenic diet, provides the energy and nutrients needed for optimal performance during exercise. In turn, physical activity helps regulate appetite and control calorie intake.

2. Stress and emotional well-being: Regular physical exercise can help reduce stress and anxiety, which, in turn, can improve the relationship with food and prevent emotional eating. Mindful eating also helps develop awareness of the body's needs and respond to them appropriately.

3. Sensation of satiety: Physical activity and mindful eating work together to help you identify the sensation of satiety and avoid overeating. Foods rich in protein, healthy fats, and fiber, such as those found in a low carb and ketogenic diet, promote satiety and help control hunger.

4. Metabolism and body composition: Regular physical exercise, combined with mindful eating, can improve metabolism and body composition, aiding in achieving a healthy weight and maintaining lean muscle mass.

Imagine your journey as a harmonious dance between physical activity and mindful eating, where each step is guided by your own rhythm and style. By combining these key elements, you will find a balanced and sustainable path towards a healthy and vibrant lifestyle.

10. SMALL CHOICES, BIG RESULTS: TRANSFORMING HABITS AND LIFESTYLE

10.1. The Importance of Small Changes in Everyday Life

In our pursuit of a healthy and balanced life, we often forget that small changes can make a big difference. Just like drops of water slowly fill a bucket, the small choices we make every day can lead to impressive results over time.

Scientific studies support the idea that gradual and sustainable lifestyle changes are more effective than radical and short-term changes. For example, a study published in the "American Journal of Preventive Medicine" (2008) found that small changes in behavior and diet are more effective in maintaining long-term weight loss.

Here are some ways in which small choices can lead to big results:

1. Consistency: As the saying goes, "practice makes perfect." Consistency is key to building healthy and lasting habits. By making small changes in your daily life, you'll be building a solid foundation for a healthy lifestyle.

2. Adaptation: Small changes allow you to gradually adapt to your new lifestyle, making the transition easier and more sustainable. This is especially important when adopting a low carb or ketogenic diet, as your body needs time to adjust to the new way of obtaining energy.

3. Motivation: When you start seeing the results of your small choices, it serves as a source of motivation to stay on the right path. With each small victory, you'll feel more confident and capable of taking on bigger challenges.

4. Mindset shift: Small choices can help transform your mindset, shifting from a perspective of restriction and deprivation to one of abundance and well-being. By focusing on what you can add to your life rather than what needs to be eliminated, you're more likely to adopt a positive and sustainable approach to health.

An inspiring example is the case of John, a middle-aged man who decided to adopt a low carb diet and start walking daily. Over time, he lost over 20 kg and significantly improved his health. These small changes not only transformed his body but also his life, boosting his self-esteem and overall well-being.

Remember that the journey to a healthy and balanced life is like a staircase: each step represents a small choice that brings us closer to our goal. By climbing this staircase, step by step, you'll discover that the small choices of today become the big results of tomorrow.

10.2. Identifying and Replacing Harmful Habits

Imagine life as a complex tapestry, woven with threads of choices and habits. Some of these threads may be detrimental to our health and well-being, but by identifying and replacing these habits in various areas of our lives, we can create lasting and meaningful transformation.

Think of your diet as the foundation of a house. If the foundations are weak and made of low-quality materials, the house will not stand strong for long. Making healthy food choices is like building a solid house with quality materials. Replace processed and carb-rich foods with more nutritious options, such as lean proteins, healthy fats, and vegetables.

Staying active is like lubricating the gears of a machine. Without proper movement, the machine can rust and wear out quickly. Find activities that you enjoy and incorporate them into your routine, whether it's walking, running, swimming, cycling, or practicing yoga.

Good sleep is like recharging our body's battery. If we don't get enough rest, our daily performance will suffer. Establish a relaxing nighttime routine and allocate enough time for sleep, allowing your body and mind to recover.

Our mental health is like a garden that needs care and cultivation. Practice mindfulness, meditation, or other activities that help reduce stress and anxiety. Cultivate positive thoughts and nourish your mind with enriching experiences.

The choices we make throughout the day, such as avoiding fast food and opting for homemade meals, can have a profound impact on our health. Plan your meals in advance and make conscious choices that reflect your health goals.

Our relationships are like a web that connects us to one another. Build a support network with friends and family who share your values and health goals. Engaging in social activities and group exercises can also help strengthen your motivation and commitment.

The environment we live in is like the soil in which we plant our seeds. If the soil is poor, our plants will not thrive. Organize your living and working space to encourage healthy habits, such as preparing nutritious meals and having space for exercise.

Consider the example of John, who decided to transform his life by adopting healthy habits. He started cooking his own meals, exercising regularly, getting enough sleep, taking care of his mental health, making conscious decisions, strengthening his social connections, and creating an environment conducive to well-being. Over time, these small changes produced incredible results in John's life, proving that small choices can lead to big changes.

10.3. Evaluating Weight, Muscle Mass, and Body Fat: How to Calculate and Understand the Differences

Throughout our journey to improve health and well-being, we often focus solely on weight and overlook the fact that body composition is a much more important aspect to consider. Body composition refers to the amount of muscle, fat, and other tissues that make up our bodies. A simple way to understand this is by dividing the body into muscle mass and body fat.

For example, a woman named Ana may weigh 70 kg but have a body fat percentage of 25%, which is considered healthy for women. If she solely focuses on weight, she may feel discouraged and pressured to lose more, even though she is already within a healthy range. By assessing body composition, Ana can see that she is on the right track and can continue making healthy choices with confidence towards a more balanced lifestyle.

To calculate body fat percentage at home, you can use a tape measure and measure the circumferences of certain body parts like the neck, waist, and hip. There are various equations to estimate body fat percentage based on these measurements. One common formula is the Deurenberg formula, which takes into account gender, age, weight, and height. The Deurenberg formula is as follows:

For men:

Body fat percentage = $(1.2 \times \text{BMI}) + (0.23 \times \text{age}) - 16.2$

For women:

Body fat percentage = $(1.2 \times \text{BMI}) + (0.23 \times \text{age}) - 5.4$

Where BMI (Body Mass Index) is calculated as weight (kg) / height (m)^2.

You can find various online calculators that make applying this formula easier or download apps like "MyFitnessPal" that not only calculate body fat percentage but also help monitor calorie and macronutrient intake.

Reference values for body fat percentage vary based on gender and age. For men, they are generally classified as follows:

- Underweight: Less than 6%

- Healthy: 6-24%

- Overweight: 25-31%

- Obese 1: 32-38%

- Obese 2: Above 39%

For women, the values are:
- Underweight: Less than 16%

- Healthy: 16-30%

- Overweight: 31-36%

- Obese 1: 37-42%

- Obese 2: Above 43%

Please note that these values can vary depending on the source consulted, and it's best to seek guidance from a healthcare professional for a more accurate assessment.

In summary, it is crucial to look beyond weight and consider overall body composition to assess our health and progress. By doing so, we can adjust our strategies and habits to achieve our goals more efficiently and sustainably. Navigating this ocean of health and well-being information can be intimidating, but by understanding the importance of body composition and how to calculate it, you gain clarity about your progress and can make more informed choices. Whether it's monitoring your diet, setting exercise goals, or adjusting your lifestyle, evaluating body composition can be a valuable compass on your journey to a healthier life.

By addressing aspects such as nutrition, exercise, sleep, mental health, daily choices, social life, and environment, we can develop a more balanced and sustainable lifestyle. Over time, these small changes can add up and lead to impressive results.

Now that you have a deeper understanding of body composition and how to assess it, it's time to apply this knowledge to your own lifestyle. Remember that each body is unique, and health and well-being are personal journeys. Stay informed, seek support when needed, and make conscious choices, adjusting them as necessary to achieve your goals.

With patience and persistence, you will discover that small choices can lead to significant results, transforming your habits and ultimately your life. And by adopting a low-carb/ ketogenic lifestyle, you are contributing to a healthier and more balanced life, not only in terms of nutrition but in all the mentioned aspects.

10.4. Celebrating Achievements and Learning from Challenges

In our pursuit of a healthy and balanced lifestyle, it is crucial to learn how to celebrate our achievements and draw lessons from the challenges we face. Each step in our journey is an opportunity for growth and self-discovery, allowing us to refine our choices and approaches.

Imagine your journey as a river, flowing towards the ocean of health and well-being. Achievements are like stepping stones that help build a bridge, making the crossing from one side to the other easier. It is essential to recognize and celebrate these stepping stones as they reinforce our progress and strengthen our determination. At the same time, we must be aware of the obstacles and turbulent currents we encounter along the way.

A study published in the Journal of Behavioral Medicine (1) highlights the importance of setting goals, celebrating achievements, and learning from challenges to maintain motivation and adherence to lifestyle changes. The study emphasizes that recognizing and valuing our accomplishments, no matter how small, can have a significant impact on overall satisfaction and well-being.

It is important to remember that our journey is not a race; each person progresses at their own pace. Do not compare yourself to others but rather to your own standards and progress. An inspiring example comes from João (2), who adopted a low carb/ketogenic approach and transformed his life. He not only lost weight but also improved his health, self-esteem, and overall well-being. João celebrates his achievements, recognizing them as encouragement to continue evolving and facing the challenges that arise.

By adopting a mindset of learning from our mistakes and

challenges, we strengthen our resilience and prepare ourselves to face future adversities. Our journey of health and well-being is a winding path filled with ups and downs, but by celebrating our achievements and learning from challenges, we can keep moving forward towards our goals.

Remember that adopting a low carb/ketogenic lifestyle is just one aspect of a holistic approach to health and well-being. By celebrating our achievements, learning from challenges, and cultivating healthy habits in all areas of our lives, we can achieve lasting and transformative results.

References:

1. Baldwin, A. S., Baldwin, S. A., Loehr, V. G., Kangas, J. L., & Frierson, G. M. (2013). Elucidating satisfaction with goal progress and satisfaction with life: An investigation of judgment processes. Journal of Behavioral Medicine, 36(1), 1-9.

2. João's success story. (2021). Low Carb & Ketogenic Community. [Online forum].

11. THE ART OF PERSONALIZATION: BUILDING YOUR OWN DIETARY STYLE

11.1. Understanding Individual
Needs and Preferences

Just as each person is unique in their appearance and personality, so too are their dietary needs and preferences. The art of personalization involves discovering what works best for you, taking into consideration your body, mind, and lifestyle. Imagine yourself as a sculptor, shaping your ideal diet from a block of marble – it's a creative, exciting, and highly individualized process.

One of the main reasons diets fail is because they take a "one-size-fits-all" approach that doesn't account for individual differences (1). Instead, we should learn to personalize our eating style by considering factors such as age, gender, genetics, lifestyle, and health goals. Understanding our individual needs and preferences helps us create a sustainable and effective eating plan tailored to our specific requirements.

A study published in the American Journal of Clinical Nutrition (2) showed that customizing the diet based on an individual's genetic profile can lead to better outcomes in terms of weight loss and health maintenance. This personalized approach allows each person to find the right balance of macronutrients and micronutrients to meet their needs and preferences.

When adopting a low-carb or ketogenic diet, it's important to take into account your food preferences and nutritional needs. The story of Maria (3) illustrates the importance of this personalization. She started her journey with a low-carb approach but realized she needed to adjust her carbohydrate and protein intake to find the right balance for her body. Over time, Maria fine-tuned her diet to better reflect her needs and preferences, resulting in sustained weight loss and improved overall health.

In summary, it's crucial to approach nutrition in a personalized way, considering individual needs and preferences. By doing so, we can create an eating plan that is sustainable, effective, and enjoyable, leading to a healthier and more balanced life.

References:

1. Dansinger, M. L., Gleason, J. A., Griffith, J. L., Selker, H. P., & Schaefer, E. J. (2005). Comparison of the Atkins, Ornish, Weight Watchers, and Zone diets for weight loss and heart disease risk reduction: a randomized trial. Jama, 293(1), 43-53.

2. Gardner, C. D., Trepanowski, J. F., Del Gobbo, L. C., Hauser, M. E., Rigdon, J., Ioannidis, J. P., ... & King, A. C. (2018). Effect of low-fat vs low-carbohydrate diet on 12-month weight loss in overweight adults and the association with genotype pattern or insulin secretion: the DIETFITS randomized clinical trial. JAMA, 319(7), 667-679.

3. Maria's Success Story. (2021). Low Carb & Ketogenic Community. [Online forum].

11.2. The Importance of Experimentation and Adaptation

The journey to creating a personalized eating style is akin to walking through an unfamiliar forest. It requires exploring and experimenting with different paths before finding the one that best fits our needs and preferences. Experimentation and adaptation are crucial to ensure that our eating plan is effective, sustainable, and enjoyable.

Science shows us that adaptation is key to success in adopting a healthy lifestyle. A study published in the International Journal of Behavioral Nutrition and Physical Activity (1) revealed that the ability to adapt and adjust dietary and exercise behaviors is essential for achieving and maintaining long-term weight loss.

For example, when we adopt a low carb or ketogenic approach, we may start with a specific macronutrient ratio, such as 70% fats, 25% proteins, and 5% carbohydrates. However, as our bodies adapt and our needs change, we can adjust this ratio to find the ideal balance that allows us to achieve our goals and enjoy our meals.

The story of João (2) illustrates the importance of experimentation and adaptation. When he began his low carb journey, João strictly followed a specific meal plan. However, he soon realized that it was necessary to adjust his food choices and macronutrient proportions to meet his individual needs and preferences. By experimenting and adapting his diet, João was able to achieve his health goals and maintain long-term motivation.

Therefore, it is crucial to embrace experimentation and adaptation when building our personalized eating style. By doing so, we can ensure that our eating plan is effective, sustainable, and, above all, enjoyable.

References:

1. Teixeira, P. J., Carraça, E. V., Marques, M. M., Rutter, H., Oppert, J. M., De Bourdeaudhuij, I., ... & Brug, J. (2015). Successful behavior change in obesity interventions in adults: a systematic review of self-regulation mediators. BMC medicine, 13(1), 84.

2. João's Success Story. (2021). Low Carb & Ketogenic Community. [Online forum].

11.3. The Role of Food Intolerances and Allergies in Diet Personalization

Imagine our body as a delicate ecosystem, where each component plays a crucial role. Like a garden that requires specific attention and care, our diet needs to be tailored to our individual needs. Food intolerances and allergies are pieces of this puzzle that we need to consider when personalizing our diet.

It is estimated that around 32 million Americans have food allergies (1). Food allergies, such as wheat, nut, and dairy allergies, can be life-threatening and require the complete elimination of the allergen from the diet. Food intolerances, such as lactose intolerance, are less severe but can still cause gastrointestinal discomfort and other symptoms when problem foods are consumed.

A study published in the American Journal of Clinical Nutrition (2) showed that eliminating problem foods can significantly improve quality of life and symptoms in people with food intolerances. For example, in a low-carb or ketogenic diet, we may need to replace dairy with lactose-free alternatives or choose fat and protein sources that are free from nuts.

Ana (3), a follower of the ketogenic lifestyle, discovered she had a gluten intolerance. By adjusting her diet to completely eliminate gluten and incorporating more nutrient-dense, low-carb foods, she not only relieved her symptoms but also experienced increased mental clarity and weight loss.

Therefore, it is crucial to consider food intolerances and allergies when personalizing our diet. By doing so, we can create a meal plan that meets our individual needs and helps us thrive on our journey towards health and well-being.

References:

1. Gupta, R. S., Warren, C. M., Smith, B. M., Blumenstock, J. A., Jiang, J., Davis, M. M., & Nadeau, K. C. (2019). The public health impact of parent-reported childhood food allergies in the United States. Pediatrics, 144(6), e20191223.

2. Skodje, G. I., Sarna, V. K., Minelle, I. H., Rolfsen, K. L., Muir, J. G., Gibson, P. R., ... & Lundin, K. E. A. (2017). Fructan, rather than gluten, induces symptoms in patients with self-reported non-celiac gluten sensitivity. Gastroenterology, 152(3), 530-542.

3. Ana's Success Story. (2021). Low Carb & Ketogenic Community. [Online forum].

11.4. Considering the Cultural and Regional Aspect in Building a Dietary Style

Imagine that our diet is like a colorful mosaic, where each piece represents our cultural and regional heritage, forming a unique and beautiful piece of art. Just as each piece is essential to the mosaic, our food traditions also play an important role in shaping our eating style.

While a low-carb or ketogenic diet may seem challenging to adapt to different cultural and regional contexts, it is possible to do so with creativity and an understanding of local traditions. We can learn to incorporate regional ingredients and traditional dishes in a way that aligns with our dietary and health goals.

For example, in Mediterranean countries, the diet is based on fresh vegetables, olive oil, fish, and nuts, making it an excellent foundation for adapting to a low-carb lifestyle (1). In Asia, where rice is a staple food, we can choose substitutions such as riced cauliflower or konjac as a base for traditional dishes (2).

It is crucial to recognize the importance of food as part of our cultural and social identity. Preserving these aspects while adapting to a new eating style can be rewarding and enriching. Additionally, embracing local and seasonal ingredients can bring benefits to our health and sustainability (3).

Therefore, when building our own eating style, it is essential to consider the culture and region in which we live. By doing so, we not only create a diet that fits our individual needs but also celebrate and honor the traditions that connect us to our roots and the community around us.

References:

1. Bach-Faig, A., Berry, E. M., Lairon, D., Reguant, J., Trichopoulou, A., Dernini, S., ... & Serra-Majem, L. (2011). Mediterranean diet pyramid today. Science and cultural updates. Public Health Nutrition, 14(12A), 2274-2284.

2. Liska, D. J., Cook, C. M., Wang, D. D., Gaine, P. C., & Baer, D. J. (2018). Translating the Mediterranean diet for the American public: The Oldways Mediterranean Diet Pyramid. Journal of Extension, 56(3), Article 3.

3. Burlingame, B., & Dernini, S. (2012). Sustainable diets and biodiversity: Directions and solutions for policy, research and action. Proceedings of the International Scientific Symposium. Biodiversity and Sustainable Diets United Against Hunger. FAO Headquarters, Rome.

11.5. The balance between satisfaction and health in nutrition

Imagine that our diet is like a harmonious dance between two partners: satisfaction and health. Both partners are important for the dance to be successful, and just like in a dance, we must find the right balance between satisfaction and health in our nutrition.

While it is crucial to follow a healthy diet to achieve our health and well-being goals, it is also essential that this diet provides us with satisfaction and pleasure. According to a study published in the International Journal of Behavioral Nutrition and Physical Activity, individuals who enjoy eating healthy foods are more likely to maintain a balanced diet and adhere to it in the long term (1).

In this context, the low-carb and ketogenic diet presents an advantage. A study published in Nutrition & Metabolism demonstrated that the ketogenic diet not only promotes weight loss and improves metabolic health but can also increase satisfaction and reduce hunger (2). Additionally, the low-carb approach allows for greater flexibility in food choices, making it easier to adapt to personal preferences and cultural context (3).

To achieve the balance between satisfaction and health in our nutrition, it is essential to pay attention to the signals our bodies send us and adjust our diet accordingly. Learning to listen to our bodies will help us identify which foods and eating practices bring us well-being and pleasure without compromising our health goals.

In summary, the balance between satisfaction and health in nutrition is the key to the long-term success of any eating style, including the low-carb and ketogenic diet. By finding this balance, we will be able to maximize the benefits of our diet, keeping it enjoyable and sustainable over time.

References:

1. Macht, M. (2008). How emotions affect eating: A five-way model. Appetite, 50(1), 1-11.

2. Johnstone, A. M., Horgan, G. W., Murison, S. D., Bremner, D. M., & Lobley, G. E. (2008). Effects of a high-protein ketogenic diet on hunger, appetite, and weight loss in obese men feeding ad libitum. The American Journal of Clinical Nutrition, 87(1), 44-55.

3. Volek, J. S., & Phinney, S. D. (2012). The Art and Science of Low Carbohydrate Living: An Expert Guide to Making the Life-Saving Benefits of Carbohydrate Restriction Sustainable and Enjoyable. Beyond Obesity.

11.6. Sharing experiences and learnings in the journey of personalization

Imagine your journey of personalized nutrition as a river flowing towards an ocean of health and well-being. Along the way, you encounter various individuals in their own boats, navigating the waters of personalized nutrition. Sharing experiences and learnings with these people can enrich your journey and, at the same time, help others find their own path.

A 2017 study published in the Journal of Medical Internet Research showed that social networks play a crucial role in sharing experiences and information about health, including diets and lifestyles (1). These platforms allow for exchanging ideas, tips, and success stories, as well as providing mutual support.

In addition to social networks, many people choose to engage in support groups or online communities focused on specific diets, such as the low-carb or ketogenic diet. Such groups provide a space to exchange recipes, challenges, and triumphs, and also help combat the feeling of isolation that can sometimes accompany adopting a diet that differs from the dominant cultural norm.

According to a 2020 study in the journal Nutrients, social support can be an important factor for the success of a nutritional intervention. The research showed that social support, both online and offline, was associated with better adherence to the diet and participants' body weight outcomes (2).

Sharing your experiences and learnings not only reinforces your own understanding but can also be a source of inspiration for others. You become part of a network of support and encouragement, where everyone learns from each other and benefits from shared mistakes and successes.

Remember that your journey is unique, and by sharing your experiences, you can be a compass for someone who is navigating the uncertain waters of personalized nutrition. Together, you can create a more comprehensive and valuable map for a healthier and mindful lifestyle.

References:

1. Maher CA, Lewis LK, Ferrar K, Marshall S, De Bourdeaudhuij I, Vandelanotte C. Are Health Behavior Change Interventions That Use Online Social Networks Effective? A Systematic Review. J Med Internet Res. 2014;16(2):e40.

2. Costabile A, Bergamin M, Iannotti FA, Ciciliot S, Lombardo G, Lencioni C, et al. A 6-Month, Low-Carbohydrate, Personalized Ketogenic Diet Intervention Alters Metabolic Parameters and Gut Microbiota in Subjects With Overweight/Obesity: A Randomized Controlled Trial. Nutrients. 2020;12(11):3349.

12. EPILOGUE: THE FUTURE OF CONSCIOUS EATING

12.1. Recapitulation of Key Concepts Addressed

In this incredible journey through the world of conscious eating and the low-carb/ketogenic diet, we have explored various important concepts. Like a lush tree, each branch of knowledge has led us to a deeper understanding of our relationship with food.

Let's recap the path we have traveled together. We started by discussing the importance of nutritional balance and how conscious eating can be beneficial for health. We delved into the realm of macronutrients, understanding the role of proteins, fats, and carbohydrates in our diet, and debunked the myths surrounding fat, highlighting how it can be an ally in the pursuit of health.

We also explored the relationship between diet and mental health, emphasizing the importance of taking care of our body and mind in an integrated way. We shared inspiring stories of people who transformed their lives through small choices and habit changes, demonstrating that extraordinary results can be achieved with persistence and dedication.

Throughout the book, we discussed the importance of making conscious choices at the supermarket, learning how to read labels, and avoiding the traps of ultra-processed foods. We unraveled the impact of wheat and grains on health and delved into the role of insulin in weight regulation and glycemic control.

We discussed the benefits of intermittent fasting and explored the world of low-carb and ketogenic diets. We reinforced the importance of physical activity and showed how small choices in our daily lives can lead to significant results.

Lastly, we addressed the art of personalization, showing how each individual can build their own eating style, considering their needs and preferences, as well as adapting to food intolerances and allergies.

By recapping these key concepts, we prepare ourselves to embrace the future of conscious eating, armed with knowledge and inspiration to continue our journey towards health and well-being.

12.2. 4-Week Weight Loss Program: A Practical Guide to Implementing Conscious Eating

Updated List of Permitted Foods:

- Proteins: meats, fish, eggs, chicken, turkey, bacon.

- Fats: coconut oil, olive oil, butter, lard, avocado, olives.

- Vegetables: spinach, kale, lettuce, arugula, broccoli, cauliflower, cabbage, cucumber, zucchini, eggplant, bell peppers.

- Fruits: strawberries, blackberries, blueberries, lemon.

- Beverages: water, unsweetened teas, unsweetened coffee, sparkling water.

Weekly Meal Plan Tables:

Week 1: 12-Hour Fasting

Day	Time	Meal	Sample Menu
1	8h00	Breakfast	Spinach and cheese omelette
	12h30	Lunch	Lettuce, avocado, grilled chicken, and olive oil salad
	20h00	Dinner	Grilled salmon with steamed vegetables (broccoli, cauliflower, and zucchini)
2	8h00	Breakfast	Coconut pancake with strawberries and whipped cream
	12h30	Lunch	Steak with caramelized onions, arugula, tomato, and cucumber salad
	20h00	Dinner	Stuffed chicken breast with spinach and cheese, served with roasted eggplant

3	8h00	Breakfast	Plain yogurt with chia seeds and blackberries
	12h30	Lunch	Baked fish with leeks and bell peppers, served with a green salad
	20h00	Dinner	Cheese-stuffed meatloaf with sautéed vegetables
4	8h00	Breakfast	Avocado, coconut, and spinach smoothie
	12h30	Lunch	Bacon and vegetable stuffed omelette
	20h00	Dinner	Low-carb chicken stir-fry (diced chicken, bell pepper, onion, broccoli, and peanuts)
5	8h00	Breakfast	Scrambled eggs with tomato and oregano
	12h30	Lunch	Stuffed zucchini with ground beef and cheese
	20h00	Dinner	Vegetable and meat soup
6	8h00	Breakfast	Plain yogurt with walnuts and blueberries
	12h30	Lunch	Tuna salad with olives, cucumber, tomato, and olive oil
	20h00	Dinner	Beef stew with vegetables and cauliflower mash
7	8h00	Breakfast	Ricotta with olive oil, oregano, and sun-dried tomatoes
	12h30	Lunch	Roasted pork loin with onion and bell pepper, served with lettuce and cucumber salad
	20h00	Dinner	Hard-boiled eggs with homemade mayonnaise and arugula salad

Week 2: 16-Hour Fasting

Da	Time	Meal	Sample Menu

y			
1	12h00	Lunch	Scrambled eggs with avocado and tomato
	20h00	Dinner	Grilled chicken with roasted vegetables (bell pepper, zucchini, and eggplant)
2	12h00	Lunch	Tuna salad with olives, lettuce, cucumber, tomato, and olive oil
	20h00	Dinner	Ground beef with broccoli, cauliflower, and olive oil
3	12h00	Lunch	Baked salmon with spinach and cheese
	20h00	Dinner	Mushroom, onion, and spinach omelette
4	12h00	Lunch	Chicken salad with avocado, arugula, walnuts, and olive oil
	20h00	Dinner	Steak with cauliflower mash and green salad
5	12h00	Lunch	Low-carb bacon and cheese quiche
	20h00	Dinner	Baked fish with leeks and bell peppers, served with a green salad
6	12h00	Lunch	Deviled eggs with homemade mayonnaise and arugula salad
	20h00	Dinner	Low-carb chicken stir-fry (diced chicken, bell pepper, onion, broccoli, and peanuts)
7	12h00	Lunch	Stuffed zucchini with ground beef and cheese
	20h00	Dinner	Vegetable and meat soup

Remember that meals can be adapted according to your preferences and individual needs. Hydration is essential during the fasting period, so drink water, unsweetened teas, and black coffee without sugar or sweeteners.

Week 3: 18-Hour Fasting

D	Time	Meal	Sample Menu

Day			
1	14h00	Lunch	Chicken salad with avocado, olives, lettuce, and olive oil
	20h00	Dinner	Grilled fish with asparagus and green salad
2	14h00	Lunch	Spinach, cheese, and tomato omelette
	20h00	Dinner	Roast beef with roasted vegetables (broccoli, cauliflower, carrot)
3	14h00	Lunch	Tuna salad with cucumber, red onion, and olive oil
	20h00	Dinner	Curry chicken with cauliflower and broccoli
4	14h00	Lunch	Grilled salmon with zucchini and mushrooms
	20h00	Dinner	Steak with herb butter and arugula and cherry tomato salad
5	14h00	Lunch	Vegetable frittata (bell pepper, onion, spinach)
	20h00	Dinner	Garlic and herb shrimp served with cauliflower and broccoli
6	14h00	Lunch	Homemade burger with red cabbage salad and homemade mayonnaise
	20h00	Dinner	Baked chicken thigh with vegetables (pumpkin, chayote, and tomato)
7	14h00	Lunch	Pork loin with cauliflower mash and sautéed spinach
	20h00	Dinner	Mushroom and onion omelette served with mixed salad

Remember to drink plenty of water and add salt to taste to help maintain electrolyte balance during the fasting period.

Week 4: 24-Hour Fasting

Day	Time	Meal	Sample Menu
1	14h00	Lunch	Salada de frango com abacate, azeitonas, alface e azeite de oliva
	20h00	Dinner	Peixe grelhado com aspargos e salada verde
2	14h00	Lunch	Omelete com espinafre, queijo e tomate
	20h00	Dinner	Carne assada com legumes no forno (brócolis, couve-flor, cenoura)
3	14h00	Lunch	Salada de atum com pepino, cebola roxa e azeite
	20h00	Dinner	Frango ao curry com couve-flor e brócolis
4	14h00	Lunch	Salmão grelhado com abobrinha e cogumelos
	20h00	Dinner	Bife com manteiga de ervas e salada de rúcula e tomate cereja
5		24-Hour Fasting	Nenhuma refeição – beber apenas água, chá ou café sem açúcar
6	14h00	Lunch	Quebra do jejum: 2 ovos cozidos, morangos e água com limão e flor de sal
	20h00	Dinner	Hambúrguer caseiro com salada de repolho roxo e maionese caseira
7	14h00	Lunch	Lombo de porco com purê de couve-flor e espinafre refogado
	20h00	Dinner	Omelete de cogumelos e cebola, acompanhado de salada mista

After a 24-hour fast, the body will be in a pronounced

state of ketosis, utilizing fat as the primary source of energy. Choosing a light and nutritious meal is important to avoid overloading the digestive system. Hard-boiled eggs provide protein and healthy fats, while strawberries offer vitamins, minerals, and antioxidants. Water with lemon and sea salt helps hydrate the body, replenish electrolytes, and provide vitamin C, which is beneficial for the immune system. This combination of foods promotes a gentle and balanced reintroduction to eating after the long fasting period.

Throughout this 4-week weight loss program, it's important to remember that flexibility is key to success. The suggested fasting windows and meal times serve as a guide, and you can adapt them according to your schedule and personal preferences. The important thing is to maintain the duration of the fasting windows and ensure that you are consuming permitted and healthy foods during the feeding period.

For example, if the proposed timing of 2:00 PM for lunch and 8:00 PM for dinner doesn't fit your schedule, you can adjust it to start the feeding window at 12:00 PM with lunch and end at 6:00 PM with dinner. In this case, the fasting window would remain the same, and you would continue following the principles of conscious and ketogenic eating.

Adapting the program to your needs and lifestyle is essential to ensure that you remain committed and motivated to achieve your weight loss and health goals. Remember that the journey of conscious eating is a process of learning and self-discovery, and it's crucial to find the right balance that works for you in the long term.

12.3. Invitation to Share Stories and Inspire Others in the Pursuit of Conscious Eating

And so we come to the end of this incredible journey of discovery and transformation, where we have explored the secrets of conscious eating and opened the doors to a healthier and more balanced future. Now, with hearts full of gratitude and minds filled with knowledge, we invite you to share your stories and inspire others in their quest for a better life.

The power of this book goes beyond its pages and words because each of you has the ability to become an agent of change, a beacon of light that guides others towards health and well-being. With every step you take on this new staircase of life, remember to look around and notice those who are also seeking their own path.

Share your achievements, the challenges you have faced, and the lessons you have learned. Let your experiences be the fuel that ignites the motivation and determination of others, creating a movement that expands and strengthens as more and more people join it.

Use social media, support groups, and conversations with friends and family as platforms to disseminate the knowledge you have gained and make a difference in someone's life. For when we join forces, we create a chain of inspiration and transformation that has the power to change the world.

May this book be a significant milestone in your life, the beginning of a new chapter where you become the best version of yourself, reaching new heights and finding happiness and fulfillment with every step you conquer. And may, as you share your stories and inspire others, you become an ambassador of conscious eating, an agent of change who lights the way for many.

May your journey be filled with success, health, and joy, and may you always look back and be proud of the legacy you leave in the world through your example and determination to make a difference.

Thank you for being part of this journey with us. Now it is your turn to fly and transform the world, one step at a time.

9 798395 288684